D1055481

PRAYERS FOR EXPECTANT MOTHERS

Celebrating the Miracle of Life

By
Angela Thomas Guffey

Honor Books
Tulsa, Oklahoma

2nd Printing

Prayers for Expectant Mothers:
Celebrating the Miracle of Life
ISBN 1-56292-538-5
Copyright © 1998 by Angela Thomas Guffey
P.O. Box 150608
Nashville, Tennessee 37215

Published by Honor Books
P.O. Box 55388
Tulsa, Oklahoma 74155

For
Taylor Alexandra
Grayson Thomas
William Joseph
and
Anna Grace Nicole

the answers to my expectant prayers

ACKNOWLEDGMENTS

There are a few people in my life who have believed in me beyond reason. From them I have known the purest love on this earth. I would like to thank my husband, Paul, for his unwavering commitment to me; my children for their tender devotion; my parents, Joe and Novie Thomas, for living goodness and giving laughter; and to Jerry and Carlye Arnold for loving me as their own. You are each one my treasure.

Thanks to my kindred spirit, Nicole Johnson, for giving wings to this book; Robert Wolgemuth and Mike Hyatt for their confidence in my writing and hard work on my behalf; Honor Books and my editor, Rebecca Currington, for partnering with me in the effort to love expectant moms through prayer.

Thanks to my Tuesday night Bible study in Nashville; my brothers, Craig and JT; my sisters in motherhood: Kim Thomas, Michele Pelton, Laura Johnson, Becky Dominey, and Carla Sam; my awesome obstetricians, Dr. Sharon Piper of Nashville and Dr. Theresa Carducci of Orlando; and a special thanks to the godly men who have forever changed the way I view God: Howard Hendricks, Jim Smith, Dennis Larkin, and Scotty Smith. You have graced me, and I bless you all.

Father God, thank You for this book. I am humbled by the opportunity to write. Thank You for choosing the most weary, exhausting time of my life to give me one of the biggest projects of my life. I can forever testify that anything good in this work has come only by Your hand. May these prayers and the intention of my heart bring You glory.

INTRODUCTION

I have come to believe that "the glow" of a pregnant woman comes entirely from the presence of God. God does not begin the work of creating and then leave. I believe that He remains and indwells the heart, soul, and body of a woman with an extra measure of His presence. Every woman is visited by the Creator God as He quietly performs the miracle of life. And like the city on a hill, the light of the Father cannot be hidden.

People see it in our eyes. They want to touch where God is working. They want to know about the new life that He has begun. Strangers see the light and are drawn to us. The world continues to marvel at the wonder of conception, reproduction, and birth—the wonder of God.

I offer to you my prayers, in hopes that as you pray throughout your pregnancy, our awesome God will come alongside you and minister to your soul. May you rejoice in His goodness and rest in His tender mercies. May you know Him intimately as friend and come to worship Him as Almighty. Press on my sister. This season will pass quickly, and the blessing that awaits you is breathtaking.

Drink deeply from these days . . . pray without ceasing . . . and marvel.

Angela Thomas Guffey

CONTENTS

Prayers

Waiting to Know. 10

Thank You 12

God Shouts 14

Rest for the Weary 16

A Peaceful Countenance 18

In the Womb 20

Miscarriage Fears 22

Many Tears 24

Blessed Sleep 26

Do Not Worry 28

My Husband, a Father 30

A Pregnant Friend 32

The Glow 34

The Heartbeat. 36

Cravings 38

Good and Perfect Gifts. 40

A Household of Faith. 42

How Many Children?. 44

Strange Teaching 46

A Disabled Child 48

Baby Stuff. 50

A Faint Heart 52

Complaining 54

Renewed Strength. 56

A Time to Forgive. 58

The Next Generation 60

A Journal 62

My Husband, My Friend 64

The Leap Within. 66

Confused By Pregnancy. 68

Our Baby's Name. 70

Feelings of Inadequacy. 72

A Crooked Generation. 74

That She Would Believe 76

My Sin 78
A Kindred Spirit 80
Baby Jasmine 82
A Godly Heritage 84
Thy Will Be Done 86
Friends Forever 88
The Ultrasound 90
Nursing 92
Guard My Mouth 94
The Fruit of My Spirit 96
Baby-in-law 98
Everyone Else's Story 100
Faith Journey 102
My Child's Will 104
Weak Days 106
No Movement 108
The Encourager 110
A Retreat 112
A Nursery Blessing 114
My Grumpy Self 116
My Church 118
A Mommy Mentor 120
My Husband, My Love 122
A House Blessing 124
Guardian Angels 126
Fear of the Pain 128
Prayers of the Faithful 130
My Doctor 132
Ready to Mommy 134
Great with Child 136
Much Advice about Everything 138
God of All Comfort 140
Baby's Purpose 142
For Those Who Still Wait 144
Forgetful 146

My Blessings. 148
The Commotion Inside 150
Grandma Helene 152
Encourage One Another 154
Confident in Christ 156
The Gift of a Child. 158
Joy in the Trials 160
Simplify 162
Baby Shower. 164
Restless Sleep 166
Be Still 168
Preview Contractions 170
Treasure to Ponder. 172
Due Date Anxiety. 174
Building a Nest 176
Fear in the Last Days 178
My Aching Body. 180
Help from Heaven 182
The End Times 184
A Baby Dedication 186
Fear of Cesarean. 188
Are You Still Here? 190
The Plan to Induce. 192
Here We Go! 194
The Time Has Come 196
We Did It! 198
A Grateful Heart. 200

Scripture Index. 203

About the Author 207

WAITING TO KNOW

MY CREATOR GOD,

Has my body become a vessel for new creation? Have You already begun to work in secret? Have You already breathed life into a tiny new being? Someone You have known forever? Someone whose days are just beginning?

I am so ready to know. Time drags by. Patience eludes me. I don't feel any different. No heavy place in my tummy. No twinges or tingles. No sure sign that I'm pregnant, but my heart is eager with anticipation. My mind races. My spirit yearns. Soon . . . soon I will know if You have been working where I can't see, knitting together the frame of a child who resembles us and bears Your image.

The thought is almost too great to stay in my head: A really big God with a really big plan for a world full of children. Each one designed uniquely and purposefully. Each one loved immeasurably. Each one known before time. And one—one precious, thought-about, already-loved, planned-by-God, living person, beginning within me. What a gracious privilege. Oh, I hope so . . . I want so . . . *please,* let it be so.

I wonder . . . if You work on Your plans in secret, then what else are You doing in places I can't see, for Your glory and my pleasure? Oh God, sustain my faith on these weak days. Affirm Your love for me. Give me patience beyond what I can muster. I know that where I can see, no faith is required. God, You know I can't see beyond this moment. So much faith is needed. I ask You to lavish Your faith on this Your daughter. I love You.

AMEN

For you created my inmost being; you knit me together in my mother's womb. I praise you because I am fearfully and wonderfully made; your works are wonderful, I know that full well. My frame was not hidden from you when I was made in the secret place. When I was woven together in the depths of the earth, your eyes saw my unformed body. All the days ordained for me were written in your book before one of them came to be.

— Psalm 139:13–16

11

THANK YOU

DEAR GOD OF MY PRAISE,

Thank You! Thank You! Thank You for this test that says I'm pregnant. I am immediately overwhelmed. My mind is racing, trying to comprehend *I'm pregnant,* but my heart is beating so loud I can't think. How can a million incredible things run through my mind at the same time? *My husband. Our family. A nursery. Names. Maternity clothes. Morning sickness.* I must be delirious with delight. I feel dazed, but I want to dance. I am smiling with You and laughing out loud.

What a privilege to rejoice with You before I share this news with anyone else. I do praise You for this extraordinary gift. All of my inmost being praises Your holy and sovereign name. May this tiny baby even praise You from my womb. You are such a gracious Father.

I can't wait to tell Paul. He has asked me everyday for a week, "Do you think we're pregnant yet?" I can't wait to dance with him and cry with him and celebrate this wonderful news. We'll begin to dream together. We'll make plans and count the days, trying to figure out a due date. We'll call all our family and ask them to join in celebrating this blessing. The possibilities are endless.

Oh . . . here come the tears . . . tears of thanksgiving . . . sweet tears of joy. A baby is the longing of our hearts and the answer to so many of our prayers. Thank You, Father. Bigger words won't seem to come, but my heart pounds out *thank You*, again and again. I bless You, God.

AMEN

Praise the LORD, O my soul; all my inmost being, praise his holy name.
— Psalm 103:1

GOD SHOUTS

FAITHFUL FATHER,

I have always believed that You have a plan for my life, but today I am captured by that truth. Confirmation of this pregnancy was almost like hearing You shout, "See, I really do have a plan for you, and here is the next important part. Rest securely, my daughter, for your life and your future are in My hands."

God, forgive me for the days I believed half-heartedly. I have moped and questioned, whined and wondered. My trust has wavered. I regret the days I have spent apart from You, doubting Your timing and Your methods. I regret that I wondered if You had forgotten about me.

You have taken my monotonous days and filled them with joy and anticipation. My vigor is renewed. I am full of the blessing of Your favor. I want to sing out-loud, pray out-loud, and tell anyone who will listen that You have done this wonderful thing. You were faithful, even while I wandered. You never swayed from Your purpose, even when I stumbled. You bestowed blessing—Your blessing, even to a blind believer like me.

Help me to mark this time as a monument to Your lovingkindness and plans on my behalf. Give me a strong remembrance of these days to hold in my heart. When the weary days come and I feel like You are being quiet, I want to look back and remember when You shouted.

Glorify Yourself through me and through my baby. A child who will forever remind me to place my hope for the future entirely with You. You are a faithful God. Your promises are sure. Your plans are steadfast. You deserve all my praise.

AMEN

"For I know the plans I have for you," declares the LORD, "plans to prosper you and not to harm you, plans to give you hope and a future."
— Jeremiah 29:11

REST FOR THE WEARY

SWEET JESUS,

I need the rest that You offer. My energy has suddenly drained. The thrill of being pregnant is still in my heart, but my newly-tired body can't seem to respond. I feel like I've been swallowed by fatigue. My muscles are limp. My eyes are so heavy. Night passed too quickly. Now, the day is before me and I have so little to give.

My burdens are the same ones I wrestle with each week, but this week I concede to their power. The laundry, yuck the laundry. Grocery shopping. Ironing. Carpool. Meals. Baths. Every corner needs cleaning. And when it's finished the whole thing over again. I'm defeated before I've begun. Where is that person who can do all things in Christ? Where is the overcomer? Where is the conqueror? Where is the warrior? I'm afraid the warrior wants to take a nap. And so, I come to You.

I want to trade my yoke for Yours and learn from You. Please teach me, Lord. Teach me about the grace I need for this season—an extra measure. You are not frustrated by my lack of accomplishment. You are pleased with the growing child inside me. Give me peace enough to receive the rest You give, grace enough to let my chores linger, and wisdom enough to glimpse the eternal.

I know full well that there will be many more days like this. But I want to be faithful to run to You and receive the yoke of Your rest for my body and soul. By the yoke of Jesus, there is rest.

AMEN

Come to me, all you who are weary and burdened, and I will give you rest. Take my yoke upon you and learn from me, for I am gentle and humble in heart, and you will find rest for your souls. For my yoke is easy and my burden is light.
— Matthew 11:28–30

17

A PEACEFUL COUNTENANCE

GRACIOUS LORD,

Grant my prayer and give peace to my countenance. Give rest to my spirit. Bring composure and still days. A God-possessed heart. A Spirit-controlled mind. My mother believes that a woman's disposition during pregnancy affects the disposition of the baby. I am inclined to agree. How could it not? Surely the baby can sense the difference between stress and serenity.

For my baby, for my husband, for my family, and for myself, I desire tranquillity and calm. I know it will have to be God-given, because our world is more akin to chaos. Just maintaining the daily life requirements for all of us is a huge juggling act. Compound that with schedules, deadlines, and homework, and we are forced to keep moving. It's a race that can trample even the swift and courageous. Even the good things, the things that are healthy and right, can add to our tension and pressures.

Dear God, speak a benediction into my life and into my husband's life. Cover us with Your blessing, the blessing of Aaron to the Israelites. Please keep me still, at least in my heart. Simplify where there is over-indulgence. Correct my misguided priorities. Restore the quietness of my time with You. Let Your face shine on me. Be gracious with my weak places. And most of all, give me peace.

There is great assurance in knowing that I am Your beloved, the object of Your favor and passion. I determine to rest in the shadow of Your countenance. I invoke Your name, Worthy God, and trust in the power of Your blessing.

AMEN

The LORD bless you, and keep you; the LORD make His face shine on you, And be gracious to you; the LORD lift up His countenance on you, And give you peace.

— Numbers 6:24–26 NAS

19

IN THE WOMB

MY LORD AND REDEEMER,

Inside me is a sanctuary where You abide. Inside my womb You fashion our child and define every feature. The thought of Your work is more than I can comprehend, and yet, I delight in knowing that You are here. I have seen pictures of babies in the womb, and I am amazed at Your work. My child at each stage of development is such a marvel.

I smile to learn that the first organ to function is the heart. Would a lesser designer have begun with the brain? And so, I ask for my baby, that its heart will be perfect. Four flawless chambers beating in perfect sync. From there I envision the rest of the body that has just begun: spinal cord, lungs, and brain. Oh Lord, our Creator, please complete each detail with precision and strength.

As the face and limbs begin to form, please grow sturdy bones and sound muscles. Make her eyes much stronger than mine. Give this dear little one ears that will hear for a lifetime. Give her a strong mind that will serve as an oasis for truth and wisdom. Lord, please oversee my baby's growth. Give our child legs to run and arms to hug. Fashion hands that are skillful, yet loving. I trust You to provide all that is needed.

Remember my baby until she's complete. Keep her safe inside until her time is appointed. I have faith because You are the maker of all, You stretched out the heavens, and spread out the earth. Your presence gives me peace. I will wait patiently while You work.

AMEN

This is what the LORD says—your Redeemer,
who formed you in the womb: I am the LORD,
who has made all things, who alone stretched out
the heavens, who spread out the earth by myself.
— Isaiah 44:24

MISCARRIAGE FEARS

LORD OF MY HOPE,

We are expecting again and I am so grateful, yet I come to You because my heart hesitates. My emotions have become worn and frayed. The mountaintop joy of knowing I'm pregnant has twice been shattered by the sadness of miscarriage. And now, to be pregnant a third time, well, I'm elated but reluctant to celebrate. One minute I'm dreaming about our child, and the next minute, I'm swallowed up by fear.

Now we wait for the days to pass and for the doctor to proclaim that our baby's okay. These days are hard, even agonizing at times. I feel like I've been on a spiritual roller coaster. Some days I can wait patiently and other days, I'm restless and anxious. I walk in confidence for a while and then I crumble under the weight our past disappointments. I must continuously surrender my worries and fall into Your mercy. Show me what it means to abide in You.

These last months have taught me that You alone are the giver and sustainer of creation. We think that we can plan and orchestrate conception, but You are the only one who can truly ordain life. And so we will wait in hope for You. We will rejoice in Your unfailing love for us. We will trust in Your wisdom and plan.

Please give me the ability to carry this child. Touch my womb with an extra measure of strength and fortitude. I pray that this time our joy would be made complete. Carry us through the wait for our precious child. Because our hope rests in Your unfailing love, I pray in the strong name of Christ.

AMEN

> But the eyes of the LORD are on those who fear him, on those whose hope is in his unfailing love . . . . We wait in hope for the LORD; he is our help and our shield. In him our hearts rejoice, for we trust in his holy name. May your unfailing love rest upon us, O LORD, even as we put our hope in you.
>
> — Psalm 33:18, 20–22

Many Tears

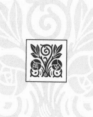

Oh Father,

How does a strong and confident woman unexpectedly become so fragile and broken? I feel as if I have shattered into a thousand pieces. My emotions have taken over and my mind can't regain control. The tears that began as a drizzle have become a torrent that I can't restrain. I am long past knowing why I began to cry. There is no reason, and there is every reason. Nothing is wrong, and everything is wrong.

I want to be held, but I don't want anyone near me. I want to explain, but I can only babble and wail. I want to run away, but I can't get up to leave. My spirit aches, my heart breaks, and my body reacts with many tears. Is this just pregnancy and a season that will pass, or is this me? Am I really falling apart?

I feel so incredibly alone. I want someone to help me, but I don't know how to ask. Irrational sobbing isn't something you can just spring on anyone. There is no one to call. My husband needs a rational explanation for tears, but tears like these defy logic and reason. I need someone to hold me, listen without assessment, and forget all my rambling by tomorrow.

Trying to pull it all in and be tough isn't working. I've never been very good at that boot strap thing anyway. Oh, Father, give me comfort. Your Spirit can console me when no one else is able. Fill this room with peace and acceptance. Hold me tight in Your arms and love all my tears away. I will pray until You come.

AMEN

Sing praise to the LORD, you His godly ones,
And give thanks to His holy name. For . . .
Weeping may last for the night, But a shout of
joy comes in the morning.
— Psalm 30:4–5 NAS

Cast all your anxiety on him because he cares
for you.
— 1 Peter 5:7

BLESSED SLEEP

GRACIOUS LORD WHO LOVES ME,

I can't get accustomed to this need for extra sleep. I have a busy husband and a family to care for, yet my body will only function for a few hours at a time. Before I know it, I need another nap. I go to bed early, and still, I can barely drag myself up in the morning. I keep waiting for some big wave of energy that doesn't come.

I wanted to be the woman who could do it all: paint the nursery, cook great meals, spend time with my friends, serve at church, volunteer at school, date my husband, and make this house sparkle. But my body won't give me permission. My eyes begin to droop and the next thing I know,

I'm stuffing a pillow under my tummy and snuggling in, *again*.

I didn't realize I was so driven to be a doer, until I couldn't do. Labor has always meant activity for me . . . producing physical and mental accomplishments. But now, during this season, the work that drains my body is unseen. The accomplishments haven't yet been revealed. I need the sweet sleep that is due a laborer.

You know that I want to be faithful to my family and my friends, but I am so tired. Give me the courage to ask for their help and grace enough to receive it. Please remove the guilt that comes from not getting everything done. Thank you for the sleep that strengthens every unseen effort within.

And God, I'm sorry for falling asleep during my prayers. I love You.

GOODNITE

The sleep of a laborer is sweet.

— Ecclesiastes 5:12

DO NOT WORRY

DEAR GOD, MY PROVIDER,

I confess my anxious heart . . . my troubled mind . . . my meddling hands. Sometimes I am so distracted about the future. Our finances are already stretched to the limits. Now, a cloud of apprehension has moved in and seems to hover over my head. My puny heart wavers. My mind questions. *How will we be able to take care of this baby? Where will the extra money come from? Will God come through this time?*

On days like this, I look ahead with fear and doubt. It's as if I've forgotten You. I'm not resting on the promises. I've missed all the blessings, and I'm only counting my failures. I'm trying to figure out what to do to save us, and I'm frustrated by my inability. I yearn for a sense of security in this world. A big, safe, well-insulated nest for my babies. Some assurance that everything will be okay. Remind me that You watch over me every moment of every day.

Are You disappointed by my wayward faith? Oh Jesus, please forgive me. I look back and know that You have provided for our every need. Help me to remember Your kindness and favor toward us and stay focused on my call as a believer—to seek You with all my heart, be diligent about what You've given me to do, and then trust in Your loving provision. Help me to live bravely and stand firmly planted against worry and the temptation to forsake truth. I am completely Yours. I know You care for me.

Thank You for calming my fears. I love You, Jesus.

AMEN

Then Jesus said to his disciples: "Therefore I tell you, do not worry about your life, what you will eat; or about your body, what you will wear. Life is more than food, and the body more than clothes. Consider the ravens: They do not sow or reap, they have no storeroom or barn; yet God feeds them. And how much more valuable you are than birds! Who of you by worrying can add a single hour to his life? Since you cannot do this very little thing, why do you worry about the rest?
— Luke 12:22-26

29

My Husband, a Father

My Heavenly Father,

Please bless my husband, my dear love, as he is about to become a daddy. He's accomplished and strong, gifted and wise, with even greater successes ahead. I am sure he will shine as a father—raising our children and shaping their lives, building for the next generation.

He must feel many pressures from our expanding family—finances, home, and work. His time is so precious, and his days already full. He wants to balance his career with great parenting, but at times he must feel overwhelmed. Give him the steady calm that strong men possess, the ability to set his priorities, and the stamina to be an anchor for this ship that has already set sail.

A great father must be a great leader, godly, visionary, confident, and persistent—a man who keeps his word. I can think of no better combination of traits for a dad than strength coupled with tenderness. Unique are the men who know how to lead but never forget how to love.

Graciously give him the wisdom to father our children. You have already given him strength of character—now give him enough success to encourage persistence and enough sensitivity to remain tender. Guard all his days. Shield him with Your grace.

I feel honored to pray for my husband. He is good and righteous and true. I hold him up and ask boldly for Your blessings. I trust in Your love and faithful concern. Thank You for the great gift You have given me through his life and love. In Your blessed name,

AMEN

Listen my sons, to a father's instruction; pay attention and gain understanding. I give you sound learning, so do not forsake my teaching. When I was a boy in my father's house, still tender, and an only child of my mother, he taught me and said, "Lay hold of my words with all your heart; keep my commands and you will live."
— Proverbs 4:1–4

31

A Pregnant Friend

My Jesus,

Thank You for my pregnant friend. Our due dates are only a few months apart, and it is a joy to make this journey with her. I'm also grateful that she is going before me. To walk with her, restores my vision and prepares my heart for what's ahead.

It's so great to talk to someone who's pregnant. She lives where I live and talks like I talk. She has become my confidant—a listener who is living my adventure. Who else would be interested in the intimacies of a doctor's visit? How many people can I trade maternity clothes with? Who better to understand when I'm frazzled by the

world? Who else could I laugh with . . . and cry with
. . . and order chocolate cake with?

I know that she is a gift from You. It was
thoughtful of You to give me one woman who
understands my stresses . . . my anxieties . . . my joys . . .
my tears because she is living it with me. I have friends
who have been pregnant before. While their words are
sincere, it is as if the accomplishment of childbirth has
purged the details from their minds. That must be so, or
else no one would ever do this again.

Thank You for a friend to walk this path with
me—a friend who loves at all times. Thank You for
loving me through her. Please love her through me.
Remind me to be a good listener and sensitive to her
needs. Because everything good is from You, I pray
with thanksgiving.

AMEN

A friend loves at all times.
— Proverbs 17:17

Two are better than one . . . If one falls down, his
friend can help him up. But pity the man who
falls and has no one to help him up!
— Ecclesiastes 4:9–10

The Glow

Dear Light of the World,

People say that I'm glowing. What are they seeing? Is it the peace of Your presence? My soul's contentment? My happy heart? Whatever it is, I want more of it. I want people to look into my eyes and see You. I want them to see peace and question its origin. I want them to see joy and inquire about the Source. I want my countenance to testify to Your hand of blessing and goodness.

More than a pregnant glow, I want a light that cannot be hidden. A light that burns brightly. A light that can be seen from a distance and draws others in. I want a light that penetrates and clarifies. I want to be a light in the darkness. A beacon that guides others to You.

So many things threaten to hide my light. Sin. Complacency. Self-centeredness. Lord, I can be such a dim light at times. I confess that left to my own, there is no light to burn. Try as I might, I cannot muster even a flicker on my own. I am a shadowy grave, except for Your grace. Fill up every dark place with the radiance of Your presence.

Thank You for the reminder that people see You through me. May I only grow brighter and more radiant in these next months. Replace my complaining with worship. Exchange my gloomy doubts for an enduring vision. Convert my pitiful worries into righteous confidence. Abide in me. Change me. Use me. God, please do whatever it takes to brighten the light inside me. Because of Your mercy and because of Your presence, I shine.

AMEN

The eye is the lamp of the body.
— Matthew 6:22

You are the light of the world. A city on a hill cannot be hidden. Neither do people light a lamp and put it under a bowl. Instead they put it on its stand, and it gives light to everyone in the house. In the same way, let your light shine before men, that they may see your good deeds and praise your Father in heaven.
— Matthew 5:14–16

The Heartbeat

Precious Lord,

Each visit to the doctor I wait anxiously to hear my baby's heartbeat. Then finally, there it is—loud and strong and clear. The sound fills the room, and I listen with quiet elation. Everything is hushed, except for my baby—her joyful heart singing a lullaby to me. My doctor and I both smile. "Hey, there she is," we whisper. My eyes become pools for tears of delight. I'm reassured that everything's okay.

Thank You . . . thank You that her heart pounds with energy and passion. The rhythm is fast and almost like music. There is plenty of reverb and a swishy accompaniment. The sound over the heart is different than the sound through the cord. From the heartbeat, my doctor determines location. I begin asking, "What's this hump over here? How is she laying? So those are feet that have been poking my side?" Thank You for the wonder of technology.

Lord, thank You for the blessing of hearing. The joy of her heart beating is good medicine to me. My fears are scattered. My doubts run away. I am embraced by the calm of assurance. The blessing of hearing redirects my vision. For a while I forget to think of myself. I imagine the face that belongs with the heart. I dream of the days when we'll snuggle. All the difficulties of expecting seem quite noble now, after hearing that vibrant heartbeat.

Thank You for the life that grows strong inside me. Thank You for her heart that pounds loudly. Keep her safe and protected. Nurture every need. Bless You my Lord and my God, for letting me hear that precious sound. In the name of Your Son,

AMEN

A joyful heart is good medicine.
— Proverbs 17:22 NAS

CRAVINGS

LORD,

It seems weird that only a few weeks ago, just the smell of food made me sick. How quickly things change. Everything tastes wonderful now, and I want all I can get. At the end of a meal I feel myself eyeing what others have left on their plates. I just can't seem to feel satisfied. I know I need to strike a balance here, but the hunger can be overpowering.

I find myself playing games—eating smaller amounts a few days before I weigh in, wearing lighter clothes than I wore last time, and heading across the street for Mexican food as soon as I leave the doctor's office. My friends are so much more disciplined—all the right foods, totally decaffeinated coffee, and absolutely no chocolate until they finish nursing. I must be the most undisciplined, expectant mom I know. Where is my will-power?

I guess I'm feeling a little panicked that I may be falling into habits that will be hard to break; and that this preoccupation with food won't pass after the baby comes. I don't want my cravings to become obsessions. Lord, I do want to eat right for me and for my baby. Help me to find balance. Revoke my license to stuff it in just because I'm pregnant. Fix my cravings on more nutritious foods. Renew my mind. Let there be joy in the eating and common sense in the stopping.

Food is one of my weaknesses that pregnancy easily magnifies. Thank You in advance for supplying new strength for this old battle. Because You care and provide, it is a privilege to pray.

AMEN

He who is full loathes honey, but to the hungry even what is bitter tastes sweet.

— Proverbs 27:7

Good and Perfect Gifts

Dear Father of Lights,

It was so kind of You to interrupt my day with gracious gifts. Thank You for this morning; the outdoor cafe, a fresh bagel, and the paper I read from cover to cover. The weather was remarkably perfect and so it must have been from You. Thank You for the banker who smiled all through our meeting and apologetically corrected every computer error. She was more than I expected, most certainly a gift. And tonight, thank You for the husband You gave me. He took pity on my tummy, cleaned the tub, ran my bath, and then quietly shut the door as he left me in peace.

You have graced me today and I want to praise You. I feel pampered and cared for. You took an extremely crowded day and carved out moments of peace and perfection. All the books say, "Indulge yourself," but You have done that for me. Only You could have anticipated my needs and provided so abundantly. I am humbled by Your lovingkindness.

Thank You for being a Father who knows me intimately. Thank You for knowing me better than I know myself. Thank You for surprising me with joy. Give me wide eyes to see the gifts You bestow, a thankful heart to receive them, and a praying spirit to bless You. I am so grateful that I belong to You.

I find great security in knowing that You do not change. You always give gifts that are perfect and good. You always do more than I expect. Thank You, Father for Your love beyond measure. I am Your devoted daughter.

AMEN

Don't be deceived, my dear brothers. Every good and perfect gift is from above, coming down from the Father of heavenly lights, who does not change like shifting shadows.

— James 1:16–17

A HOUSEHOLD OF FAITH

GOD OF JOSHUA,

A new baby. A bigger family. The tribe is increasing, and we are thrilled. A new person will surely make our home seem more like a haven, a place to replenish and rest. Lord, teach us how to graciously say to the world, "as a family, we choose to serve the Lord."

Lord, I pray for a peaceful place for this sweet baby to grow up. From her tender first days, I pray that she will know that she is treasured. When she's older, help us to make her friends feel welcome and loved. Around this table, let us pray with the hurting and the doubting, and those who would come to know You as Savior. Bless us with laughter—roof-raising laughter. Holidays full of tradition and memories. Sleep-overs with lots of kids. Big suppers. A guest room that's rarely empty. A routine that brings security. Let ours be a household of faith.

I know that my temperament and heart will play a huge role in setting the tone for our family. And so I ask . . . please start with me. Fashion Your servant into a godly wife and mother. Give me spiritual health and a thirst for truth—a secure foundation on which to build our faithful house.

Remind us each day that our time with this baby will be precious and brief. I pray that when she is grown, she will take our heritage, continue the legacy, and serve You with all faithfulness. Because of Your indwelling, may our family be known as a household of faith.

AMEN

Now fear the LORD and serve him with all faithfulness. Throw away the gods your forefathers worshiped beyond the River and in Egypt, and serve the LORD. But if serving the LORD seems undesirable to you, then choose for yourselves this day whom you will serve. . . . But as for me and my household, we will serve the LORD.

— Joshua 24:14–15

HOW MANY CHILDREN?

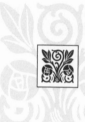

DEAR LORD,

People ask me all the time, "How many more children do you want ?" I'm not sure that's a great question to ask a pregnant woman. On the hard days, I can't ever imagine doing this again, and on the good days, I'm still not sure. While I dream about having other children someday, I'm completely focused on this child and getting it here. My mind can't begin to process the next pregnancy and the next child.

Father, help us make that decision when it's time. I do want this child to have brothers and sisters, but I easily doubt my ability. Can I mother a large family? Will I have enough love and enough time? Where will all the patience come from? To love many children well, requires a selfless woman. I know my own heart, and I have never been selfless. Please use motherhood to teach me how to love purely and give freely.

I will leave the answer to "how many?" in Your hands. I can only live one pregnancy at a time. And some days, I just barely make one day at a time. I will not worry about what hasn't come yet. Today is about this baby. I hope there will be many children in our future, but for now, I am learning how to love this one.

We will wait for You to bring peace to our hearts when our family is complete. We will listen for You to shout, "Well done. I am pleased." I'm grateful that You are already in tomorrow working out each detail. Today I will rest in Your wisdom and trust in Your faithfulness.

AMEN

Therefore do not worry about tomorrow, for tomorrow will worry about itself.
— Matthew 6:34

45

STRANGE TEACHING

DEAR GOD OF TRUTH,

Pregnancy is surely one of the highest spiritual experiences, and I am thankful for the journey. I have become more attuned to Your presence and more dependent on Your leading. The miracle of creation is becoming real to me now. I have grown thirsty for deeper intimacy with You.

I imagine that most women are struck by the same needs—spiritual questions that need answers and spiritual cravings that need attention. But somewhere along the way, strange teachings have invaded maternity. Women searching for You have ended up in all kinds of places. Crystals and astrology. Chanting and centering. Yoga and Zen. My heart breaks for those women, profoundly in need, who have stopped far short of the truth. I pray for my sisters, who sometimes unknowingly, get carried away by strange teachings. Even believers can let down their guard and be blown by the winds of deception.

Pregnancy, for me, is not an opportunity to "connect with my feminine self." It is an encounter with the God of Creation. A life-altering miracle. A wondrous event. A testimony to the truth of Scripture. Father, keep me from looking away from Your Word to account for the experiences of pregnancy. Remind me to sift new ideas through the filter of Your Holy Text. If they align with the integrity of Scripture, I will give them more thought; but if it won't push through, I'll dismiss it as strange teaching, not in accordance with You.

I give You all the glory for the truth that makes me strong. Because there is freedom in Your truth, I pray for Your guidance.

AMEN

Do not be carried away by all kinds of strange teachings.

— Hebrews 13:9

Jesus said, "If you hold to my teaching, you are really my disciples. Then you will know the truth, and the truth will set you free."

— John 8:31,32

A DISABLED CHILD

LORD OF MY HEART,

This morning I learned a huge lesson, one I hadn't anticipated. In the church service as we stood to sing, I heard a hum coming down the aisle beside me. When I looked, I saw a disabled girl in an electric wheelchair. Her friend followed behind, and they sat outside the pew beside me. I couldn't help but watch as she joined in the songs of praise and worship. She knew every word and sang boldly. After a while she even turned her hands upward and lifted them as high as her body would allow. I wept at her obvious gratitude and love for You.

My next thoughts were half-prayer and half-pain, as I realized that this girl could be my daughter.

There are no guarantees that my child will be born perfect. Our future could include unfathomable challenges. The anxious pangs swept through me.

Then You brought this Scripture to mind, *Trust in the Lord with all your heart and lean not on your own understanding.* With that thought, I knew immediately that whatever happens, whatever my child looks like, or becomes, I will love her with the mighty love of a mother. I do trust You Lord. I trust that whatever comes, nothing will escape Your careful watch. That You will render courage to the cowardly and strength to the helpless. I know that You will amaze us with Your grace.

Father, I do believe that You love me. And in the face of things I don't understand, I will cling to that truth . . . and trust. For the life lessons, I thank You. I love You.

AMEN

Trust in the LORD with all your heart and lean not on your own understanding.

— Proverbs 3:5

BABY STUFF

DEAR LORD,

I have been shopping! Who knew? There are more things for newborns than I could have ever imagined. Let me confess right now that I wanted every single thing I saw. Baby strollers, car seats, pajamas, bottles, swings, bouncy seats, cribs, bedding, high chairs, cute little outfits, toys, rattles, and books . . . my head is spinning!

Baby super-stores are phenomenal. They lure you in, delight you, confuse you, and leave you wandering around coveting every aisle. There are payment plans, charge cards, layaway, and installment loans available for anyone who wants "only the best for my baby." I confess, again, that I struggle with the balance. We do need some baby stuff, but I know we don't need everything.

When I think of how Your Son came into this world, I am humbled and convicted of my greediness. Mary wrapped her baby, the King of kings, in cloths, and laid him in a manger, in a barn. To picture the scene in my mind renews my perspective. My baby doesn't need so much after all. I had only lost sight of what matters. Forgive me; again, I have taken my eyes off You. I have looked at the world and believed their creed, "More is better."

I do believe Philippians 4:19, and I ask You to empower us to live it. You will supply all our needs. I am sure of it. Every year of my life testifies to that truth. You have always taken care of me, and I trust You to do the same for my baby. I pray, by faith, because of the child who was born in a manger.

AMEN

And my God will meet all your needs
according to his glorious riches in Christ Jesus.
— Philippians 4:19

She wrapped him in cloths and placed him in a
manger, because there was no room for them in
the inn.
— Luke 2:7

A FAINT HEART

OH GOD,

My spirit longs to cry. I am numb to the core, almost dazed, and very tired. I'm sure anyone would say, "Oh, you're just pregnant; entitled to a few 'off' days." And while I agree with the reasoning; I've become quite tired of blaming my hormones. I'm so grumpy I'd rather not talk to anyone for about a week. I just need to retreat and sit quietly and grieve my soul with You.

How does a competent woman go to bed cheerful and wake up the next morning feeling lost and alone? How did the pieces get so scattered? Why are simple tasks insurmountable today? How did the verge of tears get here and when will it go away? Who left with my patience? Is there a cure for a faint heart? I feel so fragile and weak.

All I know to pray is that You would deliver me from this pit. I have fallen so fast and so hard. I desperately need You to lead me to the Rock that is higher than I. Lord, I need the power of Your indwelling to rise above this murky gloom. I am helpless to go on my own.

I will think on Your words and pray until You come. There is no other way to overcome except by You. On my own, I prove I'm unable. I'm grateful that in all things, You understand me. I do not have to explain myself over and over. I don't have to make excuses. You are so good to accept my worn-out prayers again and again.

By Your tender mercy, there is grace for a faint heart to pray.

AMEN

Hear my cry, O God; listen to my prayer. From the ends of the earth I call to you, I call as my heart grows faint; lead me to the rock that is higher than I.

— Psalm 61:1-2

COMPLAINING

SWEET SPIRIT OF GOD,

It has been terribly hot this week and with all this extra insulation, I have been truly miserable. Now I realize that I've probably told everyone I've seen today how hot and tired I am. As a matter of fact, I've been complaining about a lot of things lately—my upset tummy, my nap deficiency, my shortage of maternity clothes, my stuffy nose, my varicose veins. I bet my friends are just about sick of me being pregnant.

Father, I confess how blind I have been to my own spirit. Somehow I have turned expecting a child into a license to whine and grumble. What my mouth hasn't said, my eyes and face have yelled. I have milked every opportunity for sympathy. Who do I think I am? The first woman to carry a child in the heat? And we have air conditioning no less. I've been so immature and childish. I'm truly sorry. Please forgive me.

The weight of Your example slays my haughty spirit. I apologize for my complaining. By Your power, I commit to turn away from my selfishness. I want these next months to be different. Lord; please remind me to bring my frustrations to You, for You are my portion and my source of strength. Shut my mouth and give me something better to talk about. Remind me again and again that these things will soon pass.

Thank You for forgiveness. Thank You that a new day can hold a new attitude. I sincerely want to walk as Your child—blameless and pure. By the strength of Christ Jesus,

AMEN

Do everything without complaining or arguing, so that you may become blameless and pure, children of God.

— Philippians 2:14–15

Renewed Strength

Everlasting God,

I praise You today for the renewed strength You have given to my body. After four months of exhaustion and sickness, I have finally begun to feel strong again. I didn't need a handful of crackers before I could get out of bed this morning and for the first time in weeks, I didn't collapse onto the bed as soon as I got home. I think I actually paid attention during my meetings, and I even feel strong enough to begin tackling my "to do" list.

It feels good to feel good! About halfway through the day, I realized that I hadn't thought about being pregnant today. It's invigorating to think about something else besides myself for a change. My new energy has brought new perspective. I am beginning to see beyond this season—I won't be pregnant forever.

Thank You for divinely increasing my strength. I finally feel like celebrating the new life inside. I'm ready to begin planning and preparing our home. I'm excited about maternity clothes and "looking" pregnant. I want to wander through the stores and imagine my baby in a stroller or a crib or a tiny newborn sleeper. I want to dream about the years ahead. I want to begin family traditions. I want to journal these days for posterity.

Let me begin to soar like an eagle and glorify You in these days. Thank You for the new power that fuels my weary body. Thank You for the power to walk and not feel faint. All of my hope is in You. From the power of The Everlasting, I gratefully pray.

AMEN

Do you not know? Have you not heard? The LORD is the everlasting God, the Creator of the ends of the earth. He will not grow tired or weary, and his understanding no one can fathom. He gives strength to the weary and increases the power of the weak. Even youths grow tired and weary, and young men stumble and fall; but those who hope in the LORD will renew their strength. They will soar on wings like eagles; they will run and not grow weary, they will walk and not be faint.

— Isaiah 40:28–31

A TIME TO FORGIVE

SWEET LORD OF FORGIVENESS,

If there was ever an appropriate time for a fresh start, it's now. It's time to lighten my load. There are grievances that need to be forgotten. Hurt that needs to be forgiven. Fences that need to be mended.

God, I begin with You. Please forgive me. There are things I have kept hidden, even though I knew You could see. Things I have avoided praying about. Places that need Your forgiveness and redemption. I have been foolish to keep anything from You. Almost as hard as confession is my hesitancy to receive Your forgiveness. Because I remember all my ugliness, it's hard to accept that You forget. I cringe under my guilt, ashamed of my sin, half-expecting Your wrath.

But You are much different than me. You freely release the sinner from bondage. You gladly pardon my transgressions. Your forgiveness heals my wounds. Your tender grace removes the scars. Your passionate love restores my confidence.

With the same measure that You have forgiven, there are some I need to forgive. There is no pleasure in remembering their grief anymore. Help me to restore trusts that have been broken. Let me go humbly to others and ask out loud to be forgiven. Let me receive their response in godliness. I want to right any wrong that might cloud the joy before me. Lord, I trust that You will go with me.

My child deserves a mother who is rightly related to You; a woman of honesty and integrity; a woman who can admit her wrongs and quickly seek forgiveness. Lord, make me that woman. By Your forgiveness, through the blood of Your Son, my Savior,

AMEN

Bear with each other and forgive whatever grievances you may have against one another. Forgive as the Lord forgave you.
— Colossians 3:13

THE NEXT GENERATION

DEAR MAKER OF ALL,

My doctor's waiting room is full of mother's-to-be—women who are carrying my baby's peers. I pray a special blessing for these who will be birthing the next generation. Their sons and daughters will make life-changing decisions and discoveries. Their children will conceive and establish the communities where my baby will live. My child will join theirs in filling the earth.

The demeanor of each mother hints at her disposition. Some are calm and pensive. Others seem stressed and already exhausted. The first-timers stare in awe at the mothers whose laps are full of children. And the mothers with children don't even seem to notice they're pregnant again. We all seem relatively composed, considering the feat we will soon perform and the life change it will bring.

Lord, I wonder if these women realize that childbirth is by Your design? Do they understand that Your very presence abides in their wombs, creating life? Will they recognize the image of God in the faces of their babies? Oh Father, I pray for these women, that at this incredibly special time, their hearts will be tender toward Your truth. Maybe pregnancy could be the catalyst that moves them to consider their Creator.

God, I pray that the reality of Your existence would impact these mothers, radically changing the way they will raise their children. Let our children know a world where more people serve You. Let godliness increase where selfishness has failed.

It is a privilege to be fruitful and multiply. It is a privilege to bear the next generation. It is a privilege to call You God.

AMEN

God created man in His own image, in the image of God He created him, male and female He created them. And God blessed them, and God said to them, "Be fruitful and multiply, and fill the earth, and subdue it, and rule over the fish of the sea and over the birds of the sky and over every living thing that moves on the earth."
— Genesis 1:27–28 NAS

A JOURNAL

HOLY GOD,

My journals—spiral notebooks with ragged pages preserve years of emotion, question, and prayer. The library of my past is a tribute to immaturity. Yet thankfully, each entry bears the signature of Your faithfulness. I am embarrassed by my young goofy thoughts, but I never want to throw them away. I wish I had written with abandon; not fearing the eyes of others— testimonies to Your presence and grace. I can laugh now at the things I once lost sleep over. You must have been smiling all the time.

The most profitable things I have written give evidence to Your work in my life. The moments when I half-heartedly prayed, only to be amazed by Your magnificent plan. The times of protection and provision. The years of silence, then, finally answers. Blessings revealed. Requests denied. Each entry has been a lesson, that I continue to understand more fully, as I recount the work You have done.

Especially now in this expectant season, I want to tell my children, with my own words, about my fears and Your peace, about my concerns and Your answers. I want to pass on a journal that glorifies You. Their stories woven through the pages. Things they could never remember. Lessons that will mean more to them later. Sweet glimpses into eternity.

May the accounts of Your presence in my life inspire my children to seek and believe. May they know of Your abiding love, for me and for them. Over and over, I will tell of Your stories. I will remind them to hope in You. I will encourage their own tender journals. So that they can know You, I write and I pray.

AMEN

He commanded our forefathers to teach their children, so the next generation would know them, even the children to be born, and they in turn would tell their children. Then they would put their trust in God and would not forget his deeds but would keep his commands.

— Psalm 78:5–7

MY HUSBAND, MY FRIEND

LORD,

Thank You that Paul and I are becoming better friends. The mountains and valleys of pregnancy can be trying, but it seems like we are bonding on a deeper level. More than ever before I realize how much I need him in my life. I appreciate him and want to cling a little tighter. I am beginning to see him in a new light.

Thank You for his increased efforts to care for my needs. His concern about my rest. His protection of my time. His new sense of drive and perseverance. The bigger I get, the more serious he becomes about provision and security for our home. "It's not just about us anymore," he says, "it's about our children; their welfare and growth."

He tells me I'm pretty . . . my new clothes look awesome . . . he couldn't live without me . . . I'm the best thing that ever happened to him. A big waddling girl needs to hear those things, and I'm so thankful he's not afraid to say them. I know that You have stirred his heart. Give him joy unleashed as he thinks of our child. Increase his confidence and assure him that You will make him a great father.

God, I praise You for this man. We have walked many paths, but this one is the most exciting by far. When I said, "I do," I closed my eyes and prayed that this was truly the man You intended for me. Now You are faithful to affirm; yes, this is the one You chose. Thank You, sweet Lord, for my husband, my friend.

AMEN

This is my lover, this my friend.

— Song of Songs 5:16

THE LEAP WITHIN

OH GOD,

I thought I felt something the other day, but now I'm sure of it. Someone is moving inside me. Bumping around, stretching and turning all on her own, my sweet baby is letting me know she is there. This has to be one of the most awesome highlights of pregnancy—the day I really know for sure that someone is sharing my body. The wiggles in my tummy are ever-increasing reminders that someone else exists within me.

Father, thank You for these gentle lessons that prompt me to examine my selfish heart. I share my body now, but these bumps and bangs tell me that soon this child will want out, and it'll be time to share my whole life. It's time to learn how to live for someone else again.

I confess that I have become far too good at being selfish, please make me better at sharing and giving. You see all the trouble spots, all the places in my character that are weak and flawed. Remove my blinders and provide me with the courage to change. I want to be in process when this baby gets here. I want to be pursing the image You have in mind. I open my heart to receive Your direction.

This baby already brings great joy. Just when my mind has wandered, she squirms and stretches, and I am freshly reminded to thank You. What a privilege to feel her jump and hiccup. What a smile the thought of her brings. This is such an extraordinary time. Thank You Father for the leap within. In Jesus' name,

AMEN

As soon as the sound of your greeting reached my ears, the baby in my womb leaped for joy.

— Luke 1:44

CONFUSED BY PREGNANCY

DEAR GOD OF PEACE,

I seem to be floating on a sea of information about pregnancy and how to be pregnant—more than I could digest in thirty years. Besides all the stuff that is written and my doctor's advice, every woman who has ever had a child knows exactly how I should carry and deliver this baby. All the facts, studies, techniques, classes, and old wives' tales are beginning to confuse me. The regular information about symptoms, exercise, and nutrition is compounded with suggestions about things to avoid, remedies that work for everyone else, and now sure-fire ways to increase my child's intelligence from the womb.

Thinking about "how" to give birth is also a complicated consideration. Do I use Lamaze or Bradley? Should I give birth at home, at the hospital, or at a birthing center? Do I want a midwife or obstetrician—medication or no medication? I have sought advise from the wisest women I know, until my cup of information runneth over, but it's difficult to know who to listen to and who to trust.

Father, I know that You are not a God of confusion. You don't intend for me to be floundering in this whole process. I need Your peace and Your direction. Speak to my heart. Confirm the right way for me to be pregnant and the right way for me to give birth. Remove my insecurities and help me to make good, strong decisions. Give me the quiet assurance that I am making healthy choices for myself and for my child. To trust You is to know peace. Thank You.

AMEN

For God is not a God of confusion but of peace.
— 1 Corinthians 14:33 NAS

Our Baby's Name

Sweet Jesus,

We are struggling to find the right name for our baby. We want a good name . . . an honorable name . . . a strong name . . . a name for any calling . . . one that would be a wonderful introduction for our child.

There are dozens of books in the stores, and we have immersed ourselves in the baby-name tomes. We have scanned the baby-name web site, checked out the top 100 lists, asked the name of every child we've met, considered *Bible* names and *Bible* meanings, sounded out syllables, researched our genealogy, and patiently listened to the offerings of anyone who would assist us. Now, every name I've ever heard has run together to become one big unattractive name. Nothing even sounds appealing to me after so much study and analysis.

Surely we can testify to this child that we have tried, really tried to confer on her a name of integrity and strength. And yet, we're stuck—confused by too much information—trying to please everyone. The world has made a beautiful decision complicated and stressful. I'm afraid we've been listening to the world.

My comfort is that You already call our baby by name. That truth settles my heart and amazes me at the same time. How could I forget Your sovereignty, even in this matter? I confess my small-mindedness. I confess my neglect to prayerfully bring names before You.

I will pray over these names until I sense in my heart that You are pleased and that we have joined You in naming our child. Thank You for Your patience with me. I love You.

AMEN

Before I was born the LORD called me; from my birth he has made mention of my name.
— Isaiah 49:1

A good name is more desirable than great riches.
— Proverbs 22:1

FEELINGS OF INADEQUACY

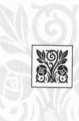

DEAR GOD OF ABUNDANCE,

You know my fears even before I speak them, but still, I lay them before You. I am overwhelmed by how much I don't know, and I feel wholly inadequate for the task of parenting.

I have read the books and watched the videos until my mind is fuzzy from information overload. I'm not sure what's right. Do babies sleep on their backs or is it their sides? Should I nurse every three hours or on demand? Pacifier or no pacifier? Cloth or disposable? Strollers? Car seats? Bath time? Everyone has an incredibly detailed opinion.

I see moms who try too hard and stress out everyone around them. I fear that could be me—trying in vain to be a germ freak. A safety monitor. A nutritionist. A pseudo-pediatrician. A make-shift child psychologist. It's scary. In my inadequacy, I could become consumed with perfection for my baby. Please stop me before I start. I want to be a balanced mother, with peaceful children and a tranquil home. I know these things are by-products of grace and mercy and rest. I surrender all my misguided efforts and confess that I am totally dependent on You.

Speak deeply into my spirit; mentoring my decisions, teaching me to be a mother. I rest in Your assurance to provide beyond what I can give. I take heart in knowing that Your knowledge is complete. I can quit worrying because You promise to be what I can't. Because confidence is mine through Christ and because You are more than adequate in all things, I pray in Your great name.

AMEN

Not that we are adequate in ourselves to consider anything as coming from ourselves, but our adequacy is from God.
— 2 Corinthians 3:5 NAS

A CROOKED GENERATION

FATHER,

I walked through the mall today and found myself staring. I noticed a group of teenagers wearing dark, eerie clothing and sporting incredibly weird hair, tattoos, and body jewelry. They were smoking cigarettes and cursing with amazing proficiency. I began to think about the possibility that my child might choose a wrong path.

Father, I know that the world we live in can be a scary place. Our child will be confronted with decisions every day—choices that will impact her life and the lives of all those who love her. For Your own purposes, You have allowed it to be so. You have called us to be in the world, but not of the world. When Jesus prayed for his disciples, he didn't pray for them to be removed from the earth. He prayed that they would be protected. In a dark and dying place, You have called us to shine like the stars of the universe.

So, I pray that You will protect my sweet baby. I ask that our family, our instruction, and our guidance will teach her how to live wisely. I pray that she will turn from the things that displease You and make decisions that will bring You honor. I pray that her life will bear the imprint of Your truth, and that You will guard her heart, mind, and body. Please keep her from the things that could rob her precious life.

Even before she arrives, I entrust her life and her future to You. I ask these things in the name of Him Who faced all evil and lived victoriously, Jesus my Lord.

AMEN

So that you may become . . . children of God
without fault in a crooked and depraved generation,
in which you shine like stars in the universe.
— Philippians 2:15

I have given them your word and the world has
hated them, for they are not of the world any
more than I am of the world. My prayer is not
that you take them out of the world but that you
protect them from the evil one.
— John 17:14–15

75

That She Would Believe

Jesus,

I know that my baby will learn about Your plan of redemption in her first few years. We will tell her the story as soon as she can understand. She will hear about it at church and at home, but it will be You Who brings salvation. Son of God, I pray that our child will come to know You personally at an early age. Please don't let her tender years be wasted apart from You.

Help us to build a home that will undergird her learning, where the life we live matches the truth of Your Word. Oh God, we pray that she would see Jesus in her parents. May we reflect the love that You have given. May we give her the grace we have received. May she come to know You as Savior, because she sees You in us.

I can't imagine the world she will grow up in or the obstacles she will face on the playground. I don't know the challenges she will encounter at school. But I do know one thing for sure. She will grow up strong and grounded, if You live in her heart.

She's not even here yet, but my spirit is already burdened to pray for her. Remind me again and again that the first place she will see You is in me. Bring me to greater maturity so that I'll look more and more like you; less and less like me. Help me to give like You, serve like You, forgive like You, and love like You. Give me Your passions to instill and Your disciplines to model. Until she believes, I will pray.

AMEN

For God so loved the world that he gave his one and only Son, that whoever believes in him shall not perish but have eternal life. For God did not send his Son into the world to condemn the world, but to save the world through him.
— John 3:16–17

MY SIN

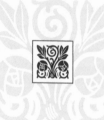

COMPASSIONATE GOD,

These months of pregnancy have become a time of evaluation. As I take inventory, I see areas that require change, places I want to grow, and most of all, sin that I must deal with. Why do I run from the truth of my ways?

If I want to grow as a woman, and more importantly right now, as a mom, it's time to deal with the issues. My heart is heavy. There's no use pretending anymore. You see all the faults I've tried to hide. I'm sure others see through me too. There is nothing outrageous, nothing newsworthy, but sin is still sin. I confess to You my transgressions—those places where I fall short of Your mark. I'm ready to lay aside all that entangles me, and run the "mommy" race fresh and forgiven.

I don't want to pass on my sin to my children. I want to begin to deal with it before they're here. I want to be growing in my relationship with You—rather than stagnant, with no life to share. I want my love to overflow from abundance, and my joy to spill out on their lives.

Lord, forgive me. Fix my eyes firmly on You and the exciting new race ahead. Set aside anything that will cause me to stumble. Point out the snares I haven't yet seen. Help me to rest in the truth of forgiveness and believe that You remember no more.

I am humbled to know that because of the cross and the sacrifice of Your son, there is forgiveness even for me. I trust in Your forgiveness. I love You.

AMEN

Therefore, since we are surrounded by such a great cloud of witnesses, let us throw off everything that hinders and the sin that so easily entangles, and let us run with perseverance the race marked out for us. Let us fix our eyes on Jesus, the author and perfecter of our faith.
— Hebrews 12:1-2

You will again have compassion on us; you will tread our sins underfoot and hurl all our iniquities into the depths of the sea.
— Micah 7:19

I will forgive their wickedness and will remember their sins no more.
— Jeremiah 31:34

A KINDRED SPIRIT

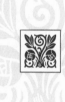

SWEET GOD WHO IS LOVE,

Thank You for my friend Nicole. She loves You passionately and inspires me to pursue great things. In my big pregnant effort, I haven't felt very inspired lately, doomed seems more like it. But after some time with my friend, I am re-fueled, energized, and ready to dream again. We seem to motivate one another, and I'm always better for having been with her.

Friendship. It's almost a lost art form. I even spent some years thinking all I needed was my husband. Poor guy—I almost drove him buggy trying to make him be my girlfriend and my husband. I guess you've known it all along, but women truly need other women for friendship, encouragement, and support. I testify to my own deep needs.

It's a joy to be with someone who shares my interests and aspirations. There is freedom in being with a sister who knows my failings and loves me through them. She embraces me as a person. There's no pretending, just gut-level honesty and gracious acceptance. It's also fun that we like the same furniture, cooking, and books. We can talk about theology in one breath and paint colors in the next. Only You could have given me a friend who is a kindred spirit.

Continue to strengthen the bond You've begun between us. Let the treasure of our time together spur me on to greater loving. Bless my sister Nicole, and bless You for the gift of her friendship. May You be pleased as we love one another with the love You have given. I pray in the name of my God Who is Love.

AMEN

Dear friends, let us love one another, for love comes from God.

— 1 John 4:7

BABY JASMINE

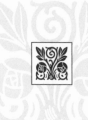

GOD OF THE FATHERLESS,

Two days ago, Baby Jasmine was left in a toilet at a theme park, only minutes after her birth. A guest heard crying and ran to rescue her precious life. She is healthy and perfect, but instantly, an orphan. My heart is breaking. God, I don't understand how a woman can go through these months and then leave her sweet baby to die?

I pray for Baby Jasmine's mother. She must be lost, misguided, and alone. Her flagrant selfishness seems appalling. She needs You. She needs to know Your love and acceptance. Please go after her and rescue her too.

Thank You for saving Baby Jasmine's life. Thank You that hundreds of families want to love her. Thank You for intervening. Please give her a home where You live and parents that will teach her about You. Show her that she is valuable and has a special purpose. Remind her that her very life is a testimony of Your love and grace.

Carrying a baby all these months, confirms to my heart that each one deserves to be. Father, care for the orphans all over the world. I commit to do more where I am. I want to join You in loving the children without mothers. Maybe because of Baby Jasmine, I'll hold my own a little tighter. I'll sing a little longer. I'll drink a little deeper. You have awakened a deep passion for mothering in me.

Because You care for the abandoned and search for the lost, I am persuaded to be more like You. In the name of the Shepherd Who saves,

AMEN

Thou hast been the helper of the orphan.
— Psalm 10:14 NAS

Religion that God our Father accepts as pure and faultless is this: to look after orphans and widows in their distress and to keep oneself from being polluted by the world.
— James 1:27

A GODLY HERITAGE

LORD,

You have given me an incredible heritage. One that I want to multiply in each of my children, but the task seems gigantic. I have always admired my parents, but now that I am to become one, I am awed by their skill and persistence.

My parents can't remember ever reading a book on discipline or child care. They just did what their parents did. They read the *Bible*, feared God, and trained us in the legacy they knew. Lord, can I do that? Will I be able to remember what my parents did? Will their words become my words one day? Will their common sense permeate my discipline and my love?

Several times in my life I remember people saying to me, "I can't wait to meet your parents. I want to meet the people who raised you. I want to compliment a job well done." Can Paul and I repeat the process? Will people want to know us because of our children? Or will they want to rebuke us?

Whatever the first steps are, it's almost time to start. Lord, I know that I have been trained. Do not let me forget my father's commands or lose sight of my mother's teaching. Bind them around my heart. Let their precepts become the light of instruction for my children. My home was a happy place. Secure, peaceful, and fun. Help us to duplicate everything good and godly here.

By the grace of my Heavenly Father, by the nurture of my earthly parents, I am equipped for the assignment. Please give to my baby, a godly heritage, one that comes from You.

AMEN

My son, keep your father's commands and do not forsake your mother's teaching. Bind them upon your heart forever; fasten them around your neck. When you walk, they will guide you; when you sleep, they will watch over you; when you awake, they will speak to you. For these commands are a lamp, this teaching is a light, and the corrections of discipline are the way to life.

— Proverbs 6:20–23

THY WILL BE DONE

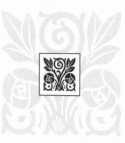

MY FATHER WHO IS IN HEAVEN,

Today I talked with my friend. Her baby was born six weeks premature and now, four weeks later, the baby's frail condition has not improved. Their eldest child has battled leukemia, and after three years in remission, today's tests reveal that the cancer is back. I am paralyzed by the sorrow I feel for this family. I know that they walk with You and trust You. I cannot help but ask "Why?" these tragedies have fallen on them.

With this child inside me, I have to wonder. *What if You call me to a similar path? What if my baby is sick? What if I give birth only to watch my child suffer? Will I be able to pray with the disciples, "Thy will be done," when it's flesh of my flesh? Will I draw from the same well as my friend, who seems strengthened by Your Word and Your sovereignty? I'm afraid to have my faith tested.* I'm afraid I won't be strong enough.

God, my heart aches. These thoughts could easily entangle me and control my mind. I know other expectant moms who have been obsessed by their fears and live in misery. Please restore peace to my heart. I offer my child to You and pray for her safe-keeping. And even in my hesitancy, I will obediently say, "Thy will be done."

For my friend, I ask You to continue to comfort her broken heart and give her peace beyond all comprehension. Oh God, I boldly ask for miracles and for supernatural healing on behalf of this dear family. Still, because You are God, I pray for Your will.

AMEN

Pray, then, in this way: "Our Father who art in heaven, Hallowed by Thy name. Thy kingdom come. Thy will be done, On earth as it is in heaven."

— Matthew 6:9–10 NAS

FRIENDS FOREVER

LORD,

Everyday, our children talk about the baby. They argue over where the baby will sleep, and who will hold her first. They have each chosen a favorite name. They lay their heads on my tummy and say, "I love you baby." I hear them bragging to their friends. They already love this baby immensely. Even at their young ages, they are devoted to one another and to this child.

God, I ask You to multiply their love. Bind them together in these early years. Create a bond that cannot be broken. We taught them from their earliest days to say to each another, "Friends forever," whenever they cry or argue. At bedtime, they kiss goodnight and promise, "Friends forever." I know that true friendship is more than learning the words, but I hope that when they're grown, they will never forget all the times they have spoken this simple vow. I trust You to remind them and make it truth in their lives.

I want this special new addition to know that family means "Friends forever." As the Lord of this home, teach us how to honor one another. Give us a love that is absolute and never waivers. Yoke these children together. Make them confidants and buddies. Disciple them as encouragers and care-givers. In a world that's crazy and often seems deranged, give them the security of brothers and sisters who are loyal and love purely.

Lord, my husband and I look to You for direction and wisdom. And we trust, that if we are faithful to pray and seek You, You will build into our children the longing to be, "Friends forever."

AMEN

Be devoted to one another in brotherly love.
Honor one another above yourselves.
— Romans 12:10

THE ULTRASOUND

DEAR FATHER,

Today's ultrasound has been one of the most exciting moments of my pregnancy. I have counted the days until we could have a peek. What an extraordinary gift to have a fuzzy, black-and-white glimpse of the work you've been doing.

The whole family got to go. We were all so eager to see that we became giddy on the way . . . laughing and pondering the baby. But the quiet room and dim lights turned our silliness into reverence. As the technician prepared to look inside my womb, we all became solemn, intent on listening and learning.

At first, we saw a muddled picture, but then, after a few moments, a hand. That sweet little hand made me cry. Then another hand and two feet. A heart that was working. A spine. A profile. A yawn. How can a baby's yawn take your breath away? But it does. God, I felt like we were looking into a holy place.

And then the technician asked, "Would you like to know the sex of your child?" I wanted to be surprised, but the room exploded and the entire family chanted, "Yes, yes. Oh please Mama, please." I surrendered to their pleas, curious myself. Besides, I knew in my heart it was a boy. The technician waited and then calmly asked, "Did anyone in this room want a sister?" Immediate tears and cheers. "Yes, a sister would be just perfect."

I will forever remember all the sights and sounds of this day. The eager knot in my stomach. The surprise of a sister. The reverence that hovered as we watched. You are truly an Awesome God.

AMEN

Your hands shaped me and made me. . . . You molded me like clay. . . . Did you not pour me out like milk and curdle me like cheese, clothe me with skin and flesh and knit me together with bones and sinews? You gave me life and showed me kindness, and in your providence watched over my spirit.

— Job 10:8–12

NURSING

LORD,

I know that I want to nurse my baby, yet I'm sometimes filled with questions and anxiety when I think about it. *What if it doesn't come easy for me? What if we can't figure it out? What if my baby struggles?*

I've seen moms nursing without a care in the world. They act like nothing unusual is happening. They can talk on the phone, read a book, or carry on a conversation. Some moms can nurse and no one notices. Restaurants and church, all no big deal. I'd love to be one of those moms, but somehow I know I'll be different. I imagine every feeding will be an event. Maybe I won't leave the house for a while, until I get the "modest drape thing" mastered. I'm just not ready to involve the whole world in something so intimate.

My prayer is that You will help me. I don't want to get frustrated and quit. Let this new baby know exactly what to do. Protect us from infections and other complications. Please let me be surprised at how good I can do. Give me patience to nurse on demand. Let nursing be a peaceful bonding time. Block out the world and help me to focus on loving my baby well.

Lord, You created this. You know how it's supposed to work. I know that You can make nursing come "naturally" for me. I will trust You and look forward to mothering as You planned. I'm a little unsure, but still ready. By Your design, I will believe I can do it. In the name of Jesus,

AMEN

For you will nurse and be satisfied at her comforting breasts.

— Isaiah 66:11

GUARD MY MOUTH

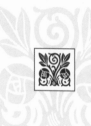

MY GUARDIAN AND LORD,

When did my mind give my mouth permission to say anything it pleased? Where is my self-control? I have taken to speaking without thinking and saying almost anything I feel. My hormones have taken over, and I'm having trouble restraining myself.

I've suddenly become much more confrontational. I'm usually easy-to-please, but now I hear myself asking that the dry cleaners redo my clothes . . . sales clerks produce their managers . . . the grocer start carrying those special items I need. And of course, my husband is bearing the brunt of my frustrations. Bless his heart; he's about to give up trying to do anything that would please me.

Where did this person come from? Is this really the woman who lives inside of me? Am I taking advantage of feeling bad and taking it out on everyone else? I don't know what role hormones play and what role my selfish nature plays. All I know is that I don't like what has come from my unguarded mouth.

Lord, I confess that I have unleashed my tongue when I should have restrained it. I don't want these next months to be more of the same. Help me watch over the door of my lips. Stop me before I get started. Keep me from harsh words and unnecessary comments.

Help me to become conscious of my temperament and moods. Pregnancy is not a license to be selfish or rude. If I have wounded anyone, show me how to make amends. Thank You for forgiveness and for the power You will give to stop and to change. In Jesus name,

AMEN

Set a guard over my mouth, O LORD; keep watch over the door of my lips.
— Psalm 141:3

He who guards his mouth and his tongue keeps himself from calamity.
— Proverbs 21:23

THE FRUIT OF MY SPIRIT

LORD OF GREAT LOVE,

I had expected, in pregnancy, to grow in my Christian walk. I had envisioned hours in the Word. Lots of time to pray. Journaling. Personal retreats. A sabbatical of sorts, to spiritually prepare to be "mommy." I'm afraid that my lofty ambition has met with the reality of hormones. When my spirit was willing, my body was weak. When energy rebounded, I battled the grouch inside me. I'm ashamed of my inconsistency.

I know that spiritual fruit is the evidence of You living in me . . . the work of the Holy Spirit in my life, supernaturally empowering and guiding. My part is to participate in total dependence and surrender. Yet, I remember many days when I took over and inevitably quenched the work of Your Spirit. I forged ahead on my own, trying to do great things by myself. I don't know if any new fruit has grown. I'm afraid that what was there may have wilted.

Lord, I seek Your forgiveness and grace. *I'm sorry* seems too trite. Explanations, too contrived. I run into Your outstretched arms. The ones that have been waiting to hold me. I cry at my frustrated self. I love You, dear Jesus. I desire more of You. This time has not been like I'd planned, but I hear You whisper that I can start fresh today.

Thank You for compassion that never fails. Thank You for new mornings. I am humbled by Your faithfulness to me. When will I learn that You don't love me more because of my efforts? You love me in spite of my failings. You are a great God.

AMEN

But the fruit of the Spirit is love, joy, peace, patience, kindness, goodness, faithfulness, gentleness and self-control.
— Galatians 5:22–23

Because of the LORD's great love we are not consumed, for his compassions never fail. They are new every morning; great is your faithfulness.
— Lamentations 3:22–23

BABY IN-LAW

DEAR GOD,

I have been thinking today about my baby's future spouse. He may already be here, still in the womb, or yet to be conceived. The blessing is that You know him by name. What a privilege to begin praying for the one who will come to love my baby.

Father, I want to pray for this sweet infant; his childhood will be so important. Please give him a home that honors You above all and a mother and a father who love each other well and for keeps. Let this child know what it looks like and feels like to live in a healthy place, surrounded by spiritually-mature hearts and mentally-sound minds. Nurture him with love and security. Protect his health and well-being. Keep harm and devastation far away. Give this baby an extended family and a community of believers who model the love of Christ. Please bring salvation to this tender one at the earliest possible age.

Bring spiritual growth and maturity for my precious baby in-law. Shelter him from poor choices and years of regret. Give life experiences that will compliment and bond with my child. Teach them both to love deeply. Let them both become believers who crave righteousness and pursue the virtues of Christ.

And when the time is perfect, dear Lord, introduce this young man to our daughter. Let their yoke be strong and unbreakable. Cover them with the blessings of Your favor. The years will pass, and I will continue to pray. It will be a joy to meet the one I have begun praying for today. I trust in You for the future; in the name of Jesus,

AMEN

Do not be yoked together with unbelievers. For what do righteousness and wickedness have in common? Or what fellowship can light have with darkness?

— 2 Corinthians 6:14

EVERYONE ELSE'S STORY

LORD,

Sometimes I want to hear about other women's deliveries, but most of the time, I wish I had never asked. I can't decide if they exaggerate, or if it's really going to be that awful. Either way, I think I've heard enough. As soon as they get into the details, my heart starts pounding, my knees get weak, and my mind begins to race. I feel myself looking for the nearest escape.

Listening to women recount their tales of emergency C-sections, episiotomies, and twenty hours of labor just about does me in. They laugh and chat so lightheartedly about their fears and reactions, but they're on the other side of it now.

I'm staring delivery in the face and it makes me want to throw up. It seems like every story I hear involves the mother being rescued from the grip of death. Just one time, I'd like to hear someone say, "It was scary and it hurt, but I never thought I was going to die."

Lord, I know if a world full of women have made it through childbirth, then I can too. Maybe they were scared spitless like me. I am not a brave soldier ready to face the front lines. I don't have any fascination with martyrdom. When the time comes, would You erase each story from my mind? Give me strength to face what comes and peace that transcends understanding. And one day, when this is long over, and a pregnant friend asks how it was, let me pass on the gift of Your peace.

Guard my heart and my mind in Christ Jesus,

AMEN

Do not be anxious about anything, but in everything, by prayer and petition, with thanksgiving, present your requests to God. And the peace of God, which transcends all understanding, will guard your hearts and your minds in Christ Jesus.

— Philippians 4:6–7

Faith Journey

Lord,

Pregnancy has become a huge lesson in my journey of faith. All nine months are about being sure of what I hope for and trusting in things I can't see. At the very beginning, I questioned the news that a baby was really inside. At first my logic might have reasoned the flu or fatigue, but by faith, I could hope for a baby. After a while, I could only verify a few extra pounds, and yet, faith got to hope for a baby. Finally, after numerous thuds and some kicks, a picture peeked in on faith's reward. A baby, yes, a real baby inside. Thank You for a faith lesson in the journey.

Now, I still walk by faith, wondering if I have what it takes. *Will I be ready to mother this newborn? Have I somehow been unknowingly prepared? Will I have enough love and enough patience? Is my well deep enough to give from abundance?* Crying babies usually make me nervous. *But will I run to the tender cries of my own?* The answers to my questions are "no;" on my own there will never be enough. But by faith, I'll press on, trusting that You'll provide what I need. Looking forward to the next faith lesson in the journey.

And so the truth is proved over and over again. Faith is never about seeing. Faith is about trusting in what you can't see. Faith is about pressing on in the Lord. Thank You that expecting teaches me lessons about the certainty of what I can't see.

The assurance of what I hope for is You. By faith, I can pray.

AMEN

Now faith is being sure of what we hope for and certain of what we do not see.

— Hebrews 11:1

MY CHILD'S WILL

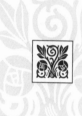

FATHER,

I have so much to learn about the nature of children. Some are strong-willed, and others come with an extra measure of sensitivity and calm. In my own family, I have already witnessed how children of the same parents can have extremely different personalities and interests. My brothers and I are alike in many ways, but we are also unique. My parents celebrate our differences, and I pray that I will honor my children in the same way.

I pray for this child that she will have a kind temperament and the strength of character to pursue her goals and aspirations. Give her courage in the face of new challenges. Let her be quick to laugh and slow to anger. Give her the ability to view life in light of eternity. I pray that early in her tender life, she would recognize the gifts You've given her. Give her an appreciation for her body, her personality, and her strengths.

Lord, teach me how to shape this wonderful, little person. Help me to respect and value the ways she will be different from me. Let me be an encourager . . . her biggest fan and loudest cheerleader. Give me wisdom about discipline limits. Show me which battles matter.

For my children, I want my love to bear, believe, hope, and endure all things. I am looking to You for guidance and preparation. Thank You that we'll get to start with a tiny newborn who will instantly teach us volumes about love. Because You love me so perfectly, I can only hope to love in Your likeness.

AMEN

[Love] bears all things, believes all things, hopes all things, endures all things. Love never fails.
— 1 Corinthians 13:7–8 NAS

WEAK DAYS

MY GOD WHO IS ABLE,

I wake up thinking I'm strong and able, then find myself weakened by minor disappointments and frustrations. Things that wouldn't normally affect me, have taken on a whole new power. I feel sad . . . blue . . . weepy.

This morning I began with a better attitude, new and refreshed. I was excited about a new hair style and a little indulgence, but one bad haircut later, all those emotions resurfaced. I felt so sad that I came home and went to bed. I know that these triggers aren't the real issues. But what is? Hormones? Somehow, it doesn't seem to matter. Real or hormonal, it all feels the same. Hopeless.

The house is a mess, and I don't care. Deadlines loom large, and I don't care. Everyone needs supper, and I still don't care. I feel sleepy and tired. I want to lock my door until sometime next year. It seems like the weight of the world is trampling on me.

Lord, this weakened part of me cries out for your power. Would You give sufficient grace to a crybaby like me? I feel guilty for being so frail. Will I look back one day and see how You graced me? I know that You carry me, even at this moment. I am helpless to walk on my own. Father, please make this all go away . . . fragile emotions . . . the guilt of my weaknesses . . . the cloak of depression.

I will keep praying that You will remove self-pity far from me. Please love me. I feel so unlovely. I love You. I need You.

AMEN

My grace is sufficient for you, for my power is made perfect in weakness.

— 2 Corinthians 12:9

NO MOVEMENT

OH LORD,

I haven't felt the baby kick yet this morning. At first I thought I wasn't paying attention, but now, after a few hours, I'm on the verge of being afraid. My mind is obsessing. My heart is racing. I can't concentrate on anything else, just waiting for my tummy to move. I've never been so aware of the stillness. Is my baby asleep? Lord, please wake her up. Is something wrong? Maybe I should call my doctor. How long should I wait before I sound an alarm?

All through Scripture, I have read Your words, "Do not be afraid. Fear not. Trust in the Lord. Always, trust in the Lord." I need that truth to be real to me now. Would You minister to my worry and dismay? Protect my sweet baby from all harm and restore those kicks of assurance. Maybe I should stop and lie down for a while. I will pray as I wait for a movement.

Thank You that prayer is so soothing. Thank You for calmness that comes to my mind and my spirit. Thank You for caring for this mama-to-be. Thank You for understanding my anxiety. In the faithful name of Jesus, amen.

Finally . . . thank You. A little nudge at first. But now real kicks. Now I'm sure that everything's okay. Immediately my fears have dissolved. I can think again. I can get on with the day. Thank You, faithful God, for listening to my prayers. Thank You for the assurance that You have heard. Thank You for the peace of a fluttering womb. In all things, You are faithful and true.

AMEN

When I am afraid, I will trust in you. In God, whose word I praise, in God I trust, I will not be afraid.

— Psalm 56:3–4

THE ENCOURAGER

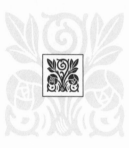

LORD JESUS,

You must have known that I felt gloomy and alone today—fighting back tears that threatened to spill. Carpool twice . . . two hours at the park . . . three red cowboy hats from the discount store . . . vests, jeans, and bandannas to match . . . fall festival anxiety . . . a nap time where nobody naps . . . three little squirts who love to tattle . . . and one waddling, worn-out mama. At the end of all this, supper could have put me over the top. Thank goodness for the pizza buffet.

It was there that You sent an angel of encouragement. After all the pepperoni, soda, and noise I could stand, I hauled my three pizza-faced children into the restroom for a sponge-bath. The angel followed me in. "Are all these children yours?" she asked, "And one more on the way?" "Yes," I smiled with my last ounce of politeness. "I've been watching you," she said. My heart sunk. I tried to replay the last thirty minutes.

She interrupted my jumbled words with, "You look so beautiful. I can't believe you're having your fourth baby. Even your hair looks amazing. My hair went crazy when I was pregnant." On and on, she went. Encouraging. Complimenting. Dissolving my insecurities. Restoring my perspective. I knew it was You loving me.

Thank You, Jesus, for the lady who talked me back to sanity—her words linger even now. Thank You for coming as a real person, with audible words, to tell me that You love me. Your timing is perfect, again. From the gift of Your filling, I give You praise.

AMEN

Therefore encourage one another and build each other up, just as in fact you are doing.

— 1 Thessalonians 5:11

A RETREAT

DEAR JESUS,

I think I need a personal retreat before this baby comes. Now that I feel like getting out of bed, my head is spinning with information and ideas. I'm reading books about pregnancy, nutrition, and baby names. I go to prenatal exercise and doctor's visits. I have suddenly decided that this is the time to learn how to sew—baby clothes, window treatments, and cute little baby quilts. Whew. I'm trying to keep up with my old life, yet I've begun dreaming and building a new one. In all my enthusiasm, I've completely filled up my days.

I feel like I need some time alone to process and pray. I need to be quiet for awhile. My private life needs an overhaul. My journal needs attending. My Bible needs reading. I need some time to relax and refresh. I need to reestablish priorities and take a deep breath.

Lord, my days are awfully busy and we don't have much extra money, but I pray that You will make a way for me to separate from the world for a few days. Someplace safe and serene. Someplace close by but still far from all the responsibilities and noise. A wilderness of sorts. I give You my request and trust that You will answer. I will pray and look for Your provision.

I'm learning about my limitations. I'm learning that it's okay to say, "I must stop and rest for awhile." Thank You for the model of Jesus, God in the flesh, Who still needed time away. Let me cherish the time You'll provide. In the name of Jesus, Who slipped away to pray,

AMEN

But He Himself would often slip away to the wilderness and pray.

— Luke 5:16 NAS

A NURSERY BLESSING

DEAR MAKER OF HEAVEN AND EARTH,

We have lovingly prepared this nursery for our baby but consider it unfinished without Your blessing. Father, we invite You to abide in this room. Dwell here with an abundance of peace and comfort. Station angels over the doors and upon each corner to guard the precious one who will rest here. Make this simple nursery a place of serenity and grace.

In this crib, we will lay our precious bundle. Give our little one peaceful sleep; free from colic and pains that disturb. Keep close watch over every breath. Let the sights from this bed be intriguing and exciting.

On this table we'll change our baby. Make us superb care-givers, with an extra portion of intuition and wisdom. Teach us how to discern what different cries mean. Guide us as we learn to be sensitive to our baby's unique needs.

And in this chair, we'll find pleasure in holding the treasure that You bestow. We will rock and cuddle. We will sing songs and begin to teach our baby about the Savior. We'll pray out-loud and sing hushed hymns of praise. A bond will be established that can never be broken. God, we pray for years of rocking and snuggles. Let our time be tender and blessed.

Knowing that You are here makes our preparations for this nursery complete—ready to receive Your gift. We look forward to introducing our child to the place where You are waiting. Because we love You and esteem You, we humbly invoke Your blessing on this room, our family, and especially the new life that will soon be here. In the name of Jesus,

AMEN

The LORD remembers us and will bless us: He will bless the house of Israel, he will bless the house of Aaron, he will bless those who fear the LORD—small and great alike. May the LORD make you increase, both you and your children. May you be blessed by the LORD, the Maker of heaven and earth.

— Psalm 115:12–15

115

My Grumpy Self

LORD,

I understand that moodiness is part of pregnancy, but these last months, I have become one grumpy person. I don't want to be this way. I'm tired of crying over very little things. I'm weary of the anger that comes over me. This is not "me." I am not moody or weepy or angry. But now it seems like I'm spending a lot of energy trying not to explode, trying to keep what's boiling inside from coming out for the whole world to see.

The worst part is that I almost always erupt at home with Paul and the children. I find myself apologizing for harsh words and a short fuse. I explain my tired legs, my heavy tummy, and my aching back. Everyone looks at me with dutiful sympathy. They forgive me, but I feel worse for unloading on the people I love most.

Father, forgive me and help me to make it through the last months of pregnancy. You understand what's going on in my body much better than I do. I don't know where these clouds of gloom come from. I can't see what's going on inside that affects my emotions so drastically. I truly want to build others up with my words, but the power will have to come from You. I've tried on my own and failed miserably. I want to commit each day to wholesome words that edify and encourage.

You are my strength when I am weak. You are able when I am helpless. By the power of the Holy Spirit and because of Your forgiveness, I pray and expect that You'll answer.

AMEN

Do not let any unwholesome talk come out of your mouths, but only what is helpful for building others up according to their needs, that it may benefit those who listen.

— Ephesians 4:29

My Church

DEAR JESUS,

I want to thank You for my church family. They have been gracious to love my family and tenderhearted toward me in these months of pregnancy. They have welcomed us as their own with an outpouring of love like I've never known before. You must genuinely dwell in their midst.

I'm so thankful to be in community with these believers. They are teaching me by example. Some have already brought meals to us, and the baby isn't even here yet. A lovely woman offered to come and clean our house as a gift. Friends have kept our children so that I can rest. A girl named Jessica helps me get our three little ones to their Sunday School classes. People have already volunteered to be on standby in case we have to go to the hospital in the middle of the night. There have been encouraging phone calls and sweet notes of love and inspiration.

These believers have truly become my family. I love them and I love You in them. Father, I ask You to honor their faithful deeds. Entrust them with a mighty work for Your kingdom. Bring a multitude to salvation through their gracious acceptance and love. Glorify Yourself through them.

While pregnant and exhausted, it would be easy to stop going to church, but I can't imagine the lost blessing. I'm not very active, but it's not time to be. This is a time of rest and receiving. All the years of doing are being returned many-fold. Lord, I pray for all my expectant sisters, that they too will know the beauty and blessing of a church family. In Your great name,

AMEN

Let us not give up meeting together, as some are in the habit of doing, but let us encourage one another—and all the more as you see the Day approaching.

— Hebrews 10:25

A MOMMY MENTOR

DEAR GOD OF GRACE,

I am really missing my mother today. All these miles apart and I need her input and advice, encouragement and correction. I need her to show me how to care for my baby. I need the security of her watchful eye. To talk is a blessing, but to be with her would be better. For now, the phone is the best we can do.

Lord, I need a substitute mother, someone who will pour her wisdom into my life. Someone close-by to take these first steps with me. Someone who loves You. Someone I can trust. Someone who has learned how to balance the demands of a family. It would be so helpful to watch a great mother in action.

I realize that I am a younger woman who needs training. To read a book is one thing, but to observe in real life is another. I have been yearning for a mother who would train me—someone who is eager to teach what she has learned.

As I pray, I will begin to look for my mentor. I will ask at my church and seek out my friends. I ask You to ready her heart to receive me. Help her to carve out some time in her life for me. Bind us together in purpose. She: the seasoned pro. Me: a fledgling rookie.

Thank You for the woman You will send into my life. Let her motivate me to keep growing as a mom—looking more and more like You, less and less like me. In pursuit of godliness, I pray.

AMEN

Teach the older women to be reverent in the way they live. . . . Then they can train the younger women to love their husbands and children.

— Titus 2:3–4

MY HUSBAND, MY LOVE

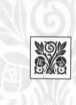

DEAR LORD,

My husband just walked through the door looking even more weary than I feel, and yet his spirit is shining. He was kind and gentle and ordered me out of the kitchen. He took over and sent me to rest. His selflessness is very humbling.

I believe that he looks more like You than ever before in our marriage. He continues to be firmly committed to keeping the promises he made to me in Your presence. He wants to love me as Christ loved the church, and I am so honored to call him mine. Thank You for the depth of his love for me. Thank You for his perseverance in the world and in our home. Thank You that I have grown because of him, and through him. Thank you that he cares for me and puts my needs before his. You must be so pleased with Your son.

Lord God, I ask You to bless this sweet man. Multiply the fruit of his labor. Clear the path where he walks. Protect his comings and goings. Give him wisdom beyond his years. Strengthen his friendships and make them pure. Give him a vision for our future and the ability to lead. Make him a great daddy.

Lord, show me how to love him with a holy love. Let our lives together be a beautiful offering, one that brings you pleasure. May our children know true love because they watched their parents. May our sons love their wives because their daddy loved me. Thank You for Paul. And thank You that he is Your man. Because of the love of Christ,

AMEN

Husbands, love your wives, just as Christ loved the church and gave himself up for her to make her holy. . . . husbands ought to love their wives as their own bodies. He who loves his wife loves himself. After all, no one ever hated his own body, but he feeds and cares for it, just as Christ does the church.

— Ephesians 5:25–26, 28–29

A House Blessing

DEAR LORD OF ALL,

I ask that You would bless this house that has become a home for our family. It has served us well, but soon it will have to stretch to encompass a new family member. I can't wait for these rooms to be filled once again with the excitement of new life.

I walk through each door and dream about the flurry of activity ahead. Family and friends coming to bid us love and hold our new one. A living room scattered with blankets and toys. A nursery that's no longer spotless. Sheets to be changed and a diaper pail to empty. A crib with a baby nestled there. A mobile that sings for its audience of one. A hamper full of tiny new clothes.

Bedrooms lit by night lights and the glow of a baby monitor. Lullabies and cries. A swing that holds more than a teddy bear.

Lord, please bless each room. Establish our home as a haven for all who live here. Build a spiritual moat to protect us from harm. Fill this place with Your presence. Give us secure walls to weather any storm. Teach us how to honor one another and show kindness to strangers. May these walls be bursting with laughter. Build this house with wisdom and bless us with the riches and treasures that come from love.

Only by Your presence, will this house be transformed. Only by Your hand will it be a special place that will shelter and protect all those who dwell within. We welcome You and invite Your Spirit to always live among us. In the precious name of our Savior, I pray,

AMEN

By wisdom a house is built, and through understanding it is established; through knowledge its rooms are filled with rare and beautiful treasures.

— Proverbs 24:3–4

Guardian Angels

Almighty God,

I take comfort in knowing that you send angels to protect us from the world's dangers. I ask that even now, You would direct angels to guard our sweet baby.

In the womb, I ask for protection. Keep us both healthy and fit until the appointed day. Safeguard my body from disease and infection. Regulate each element of pregnancy. Keep my feet from stumbling. Watch over my comings and goings. Remove accidents and destruction far from us. Let angels intervene where danger may lurk.

In delivery, please go before us. Prepare our room for safety and health. Orchestrate a gifted staff to care for her. Shelter her from unseen peril. Post angels at every turn. And for the rest of her life, dear God, appoint angels to defend and preserve. Because I know You go before her and with her, my fears about the world are in check. Every time I look away . . . every street she will ever cross . . . every person in whom she will place her trust . . . every day of preschool and elementary, high school and college . . . I ask You to be there; readying the heavenly troops, giving instruction to powerful forces, prepared and alert to protect.

I am secure in Your strength. When I am afraid I will pray and envision the angels You promise. I will dwell in Your shelter and rest in Your shadow. I will not fear, because You are faithful. Because You are a fortress for those who love You; because You guard us with angels; there is courage and power when I pray.

AMEN

The angel of the LORD encamps around those who fear him, and he delivers them.

— Psalm 34:7

For he will command his angels concerning you to guard you in all your ways.

— Psalm 91:11

FEAR OF THE PAIN

MY LORD,

I've only had a few sharp jabs of pain so far, but they're enough to tell me what's coming. I know it's eventually got to happen, but how do you ever get ready to endure the pain of giving birth? Breathing techniques, varied positions, low lights, soft music, massages—they all seem like a bucket of water thrown onto a forest fire—thanks for the try, but the fire rages on.

If there's some way to be psyched up or mentally prepared, Lord, I pray that You will help me get ready to endure the process. Provide an abundance of courage. Remind me constantly that each new contraction brings me one step closer to my baby.

Forgive me for being so silly, but I'm already practicing saying, "Epidural, please." I probably won't be able to hang that invisible, yet boasted, award on my wall. The one that reads, "This woman gave birth without the assistance of drugs." I have been spending a lot of time wondering if epidurals are part of Your plan? I hope so. I keep hearing that women have been giving birth naturally forever. People used to get their teeth pulled without anesthetic too, but who would still choose that option?

I always choose to avoid pain whenever I can, but in this situation, there is no choice. So, I will continue to pray and put my trust in You. Stamina, guts, willpower—they will all have to come from You. I know that You will provide. Every time I am afraid, I will come before You, where the perfect love of God casts out all fear. Hold me tight and love me long. I need You.

AMEN

To the woman he said, "I will greatly increase your pains in childbearing; with pain you will give birth to children."

— Genesis 3:16

PRAYERS OF THE FAITHFUL

FATHER,

Thank You for all the people who have joined me in prayer. So many have taken the time to tell me they are praying for me and for our child. Others have written sweet notes to let me know they are praying, and a little child recently told me that she was praying for our baby everyday. Please bless the faithfulness of these precious people who are willing to love my family through prayer.

I really do cherish their prayers, because I believe in the power of prayer. I believe that You hear us and that You are moved by the prayers of the righteous. I also believe that sometimes You wait to act until prayers are offered in faith. Keep teaching me more and more about prayer. But mostly, keep me motivated to pray.

Lord, I confess that my prayer-life often stumbles. Some days I put off praying, waiting for a quiet moment that never comes. Other times I pray, but lack the power that comes from faith and passion. Make me thirsty for you. Remind me to pray for all things and without ceasing. Put passion back in this tired old body, and glorify Yourself in my prayers.

Somebody prayed for me—a sacrifice of time . . . a loving gift . . . a sweet offering of friendship. I am humbled and blessed. Bond us together through prayer. Strengthen the praying and let them see the fruit of their prayers. Thank You for the unity and peace that comes from seeking You together. Because the Bible tells me to . . . I pray.

AMEN

Pray for each other so that you may be healed. The prayer of a righteous man is powerful and effective.

— James 5:16

MY DOCTOR

GOD,

I want to thank You for my obstetrician. I am blessed to have such a qualified physician caring for me and my baby. She gives attention to my tiniest concerns and symptoms. She answers my questions like I'm the first one to ask. She seems as thrilled as I that I'm having a baby. I'm so grateful for her time and courtesy.

To choose to care for women who are slightly afraid, emotionally charged, and extremely inquisitive is truly a high calling. I imagine her work to be both rewarding and exhausting. God, I ask that You would be kind to my doctor. Give her wisdom and common sense. Increase her stamina when the babies come all night. Multiply her patience and joy. Keep her heart tender toward the hurt and suffering. Provide more victories than defeats. Let the miracle of birth never grow dull.

I pray that she would look to You as the Great Physician—that she would know You personally as the Giver of Life. Remind her that she is an instrument in Your hands. Teach her to look to You for wisdom and guidance. Increase her knowledge. Astound her with the wonder of creation. Whisper that it's You she assists in delivery.

I ask that You would see that my doctor is at the top of her game for my baby's debut. Surround her with a superior staff. Let everything run smoothly. Bless all her efforts on our behalf. Thank You for overseeing every little detail. Because You are the Great Physician, I trust You to work through the one I have chosen. I rest in You.

AMEN

God was kind to the midwives and the people
increased and became even more numerous.
And because the midwives feared God, he gave
them families of their own.

— Exodus 1:20–21

READY TO MOMMY

LORD OF MY NEW PATH,

Expecting has been good, but now I'm anxious to become a mommy again. I can't wait to hold the one I have dreamed of. I'll be thrilled to push a stroller. It will be pure joy to lug a car seat. I want someone to wear those little pajamas. The room is all ready. The wallpaper hung. I want once more to rock in my chair. Nine long months of waiting and praying, have made me eager for the life-change ahead.

Thank You for the new thing You are doing in our family—for the new member You are bringing to our tribe. Thank You for the time we have had to prepare. I want to look ahead and let go of the past.

I can just begin to see the new stream in our desert. I am ready to share again—ready to give myself away completely one more time.

You know, I feel like I'm being promoted. From "mother of three" to "mother of four." More responsibility, but more fringe benefits than I deserve. I look forward to giving all of my heart, mind, and energy in exchange for the love of a child—sounds like a fair trade to me. I'm ready to start.

You are so good to bring new life to our home. A brand new person, touching all our lives in brand new ways. We look forward to all You have prepared. We walk ahead totally by faith, filled with the joy of anticipation. Because You do new things, I give You praise.

AMEN

Forget the former things; do not dwell on the past. See, I am doing a new thing! Now it springs up; do you not perceive it? I am making a way in the desert and streams in the wasteland.
— Isaiah 43:18–19

GREAT WITH CHILD

LORD,

When I think of Mary, being "great with child,"
I picture radiance and beauty, surrounded by angels
and aglow with your presence; her countenance
serene and her spirit composed. I'm sure my image
has been tainted by one too many embossed nativity
scenes, but I think of her as pure and ideal.

When I look at myself, the resemblance is
weak. I am only "great"—as in big—everywhere.
Great ankles. Great hips. Great big tummy. Great
swollen fingers. And a great puffy face. I've been big
for so long, I can't remember not being "great." Are
the clothes in the back of my closet really mine?
Have I become a "comfortable shoe" woman? Will I

ever be able to wear a belt again? Have I lost all sense of style, forever doomed to big clothes with no waist to bind or pinch? The scariest part is that some of my maternity clothes are too tight, and I still have a way to go.

Lord, I guess I'm afraid of never being the old me again. Never fitting into jeans. Never losing all the weight I've put on. Becoming a dowdy mom in sweat pants, with spit-up on my shoulder and my hair in a ponytail. I know my fears aren't very spiritual, but they're real. I bring them to You so that we can begin to deal with them. Help me set practical goals. Calm my fears.

Please renew my perspective. When I worry about myself, remind me that these days are about the baby. My time will come soon enough. "Great with child" is a blessing. I want to honor You, even in my "greatness."

AMEN

And Joseph also went up from Galilee . . . with Mary, his espoused wife, being great with child.
— Luke 2:4,5 KJV

MUCH ADVICE
ABOUT EVERYTHING

ALL-KNOWING GOD,

I want to be faithful to seek wise counsel,
especially during this new adventure. I want to
listen to the women who have gone before me and
learn from their insights. I want to study and glean
from their teaching. But, I never imagined that there
would be so much advice about everything. I feel
like I'm drowning.

Everyone seems to have an opinion, a way
that is better, a cure for any ailment, or something
they want me to seriously consider. I want to walk
through this pregnancy with the advice of my
doctors and input from others I respect. But

strangers, and people I barely know, want to tell me what birthing technique is best, which hospital to go to, their home remedies for sleeplessness, and more intimate information than I can handle.

I need Your wisdom to process all the voices who want to tell me how to be pregnant. I want to hear Your voice above all the unsolicited clamor. Let me be gracious with the givers of advice. Remind me to thank them for their interest and concern. Help me to hold onto truth and quickly release all the rest.

Watch over my mind, and keep me from misguided decisions. Let the Holy Spirit be my guide, discerning what's right and appropriate for me. My baby's health and safety are my utmost concern. Let me always do the best for my child. Because You are all-knowing, I will come to You with the advice I've been given and continue to pray about every decision. In the name of the One I trust with my life, my dear Jesus,

AMEN

Plans fail for lack of counsel, but with many advisers they succeed.
— Proverbs 15:22

Make plans by seeking advice.
— Proverbs 20:18

God of All Comfort

Father of Compassion,

Thank You for all the comfort You have provided through these months. You have patiently endured my whiny prayers and questioning heart. You have given strength to these weary bones and provided my husband with an extra measure of grace while "we're pregnant" one more time. You have provided godly friends to intervene and hold me up. The end is in sight, and I can truly testify to Your provision through the suffering and troubles of pregnancy.

I want to hide away in my heart each of the lessons You have taught me during these months. I ask that You would provide opportunities for me to use the valuable things I've learned so that others may be comforted with the same comfort I have received from You.

Forever give me tender compassion for other expectant moms. Teach me how I can best love them and serve them. Give me grace and mercy that overflows. Remind me to be a giver of prayer and time and resources. Help me to recall the fatigue, so I can give rest. Show me undone chores that I can help do. Give me compassion for teary eyes that need to cry. Use my hands, my heart, and my words to encourage and uplift.

You have given so much to me in this season. I have every reason to give back, in the name, and because of the mercy, of Jesus Christ. You have been a lover of my soul and I cherish You. It will be a privilege to be a giver of comfort, because You have been my God of all comfort.

AMEN

Praise be to the God and Father of our Lord Jesus Christ, the Father of compassion and the God of all comfort, who comforts us in all our troubles, so that we can comfort those in any trouble with the comfort we ourselves have received from God. For just as the sufferings of Christ flow over into our lives, so also through Christ our comfort overflows.

— 2 Corinthians 1:3–5

BABY'S PURPOSE

GOD OF CREATION,

I can hardly comprehend that You already know my baby. We can't even decide on a name, yet You have always called her by name. You know her disposition and her passions. You know her favorite color and her favorite food. You know what she'll look like when she's sixteen, and You even know the names of her children. I can't begin to fathom the depth of Your knowledge.

Father, I pray for this sweet child, that early in life, she will discover Your purpose for her life—that special thing that makes her heart sing. Teach her to know the still small voice of the Holy Spirit that says, "this is the way, walk in it." Give her the excitement that comes from loving what you do . . . the thrill of devoting a lifetime to one's passion.

Lord, I have spent many years searching for my passions. I struggled with what everyone else wanted. I wasted years chasing money or things not connected to what You have called me to do. It's taken a long time to begin to be okay with who I am, but more importantly with who I am not. So much mis-direction could have been avoided if I had looked for You sooner. I pray for my children that they'll know Your will early—that they will have ears to hear and a compassionate heart to respond.

I can't wait to see what she'll become. I can't wait to see what You already know. It'll be worth a lifetime of loving and praying to watch her become all she can be. I humbly pray in Your name,

AMEN

Before I formed you in the womb I knew you,
before you were born I set you apart.
— Jeremiah 1:5

FOR THOSE WHO STILL WAIT

GIVER OF LIFE,

My heart is burdened today for my friends who cannot have children. Like Hannah, they have spent years praying and grieving for a child who never comes. They are frazzled—worn out by doctors, books, specialists, drugs, and procedures. Many even dread seeing their families, weary of their sympathetic looks and tired of the same conversation. I grieve for my sisters and long for them to experience the wonder of new life growing and flourishing within their bodies.

Lord, give me tender compassion when I'm with them. I find myself talking about anything but pregnancy, overcompensating, understating the obvious, hoping I won't say something hurtful. Even so, I think it hurts them just to be with me. I know some women who can't go to baby showers or visit their friends with babies because their hearts are too raw and their pain too intense. I mourn for their hurt and pray for their healing.

Most of all, I ask that You would hear their prayers. Remember them. And grant them the answers they seek. After many years, You remembered Hannah and opened her womb. Please see my friends in their lament and answer their pleas for children. Let them rejoice with Hannah, who said in 1 Samuel 1:27, "I prayed for this child, and the LORD has granted me what I asked of him."

Thank You, Father, for watching over those who wait. I believe in the sufficiency of Your grace. I trust in the perfection of Your will. Because You bring life to the barren, there is power in my prayer.

AMEN

In bitterness of soul Hannah wept much and prayed to the LORD.
— 1 Samuel 1:10

He settles the barren woman in her home as a happy mother of children. Praise the LORD.
— Psalm 113:9

Forgetful

Dear Lord,

I know that I have forgotten a lot lately, but tonight has been the most frustrating. I lost my keys somewhere between the car and the church. They aren't in my purse. They aren't at the church. Only You know where they are. I understand that forgetting is part of being pregnant, but I'm very put out with myself.

What's going on with my brain? I'm usually a detail person, but a fog seems to have moved in and settled over my mind. I can't remember names. I walk into a room and forget why I'm there. I open the dictionary and forget the word I wanted to spell. I've taken to posting reminders on the cabinets and doors, in case something urgent gets overlooked. When I get in the car, I must tell myself over and over where I'm going or I run the risk of driving right past. I want my old brain back. Sharp as a tack. I'm tired of trying to remember what I've forgotten.

I've taken time off from Scripture memory. And I'm praying it'll all come back to me. Please, Lord, somewhere deep inside, keep Your Word stored safely within me. Restore wisdom, and all the past years of learning. And on the other side of this haze, replenish my mind.

I love You, dear Jesus, and will depend on You to take care of my lost self. Don't let me do anything crazy or cause harm to anyone else. And about my keys . . . well, now I've forgotten what I needed them for. Protected by Your watchful eye, I pray in the name of Jesus.

AMEN

Get wisdom, get understanding; do not forget my words or swerve from them.

— Proverbs 4:5

MY BLESSINGS

LORD GOD,

To you be the glory for all the great things you have done and are doing on behalf of this baby and me.

Thank you for the life that kicks and squirms inside me;
my body that groans and creaks,
but makes it through another day;
a husband who does the dishes and overlooks the mess;
children who can't wait to see their new sibling;
my church that prays;
a friend who calls and listens;
my parents who worry about their baby;
my doctor and my insurance;

little baby clothes sewn by faithful hands;

Sunday naps;

the freedom to abstain from new obligations;

the sweet sense of anticipation that enhances every day;

our home, ready to be shared with another;

your abundant provision for us;

preparing me to love another with my life;

your Son, the giver of eternal life, and the model of grace.

In the name of the One Who came as a baby, I praise You for blessings.

AMEN

Many, O LORD my God, are the wonders which Thou hast done, And Thy thoughts toward us; There is none to compare with Thee; If I would declare and speak of them, They would be too numerous to count.

— Psalm 40:5 NAS

THE COMMOTION INSIDE

LORD,

This must be a new phase of pregnancy. I can look at my tummy and watch a person moving. It almost seems eerie to experience my belly rolling like a wave or to see a rounded shape bulge from my side. I feel a flurry of activity in there. Something is stuck up under my ribs, poking and pointing around. Little toes, I suspect. My lungs are crowded; my breathing is shallow. There is a body part jammed into my back. It's been there so long I'm sore in one spot.

I've seen pictures and watched the ultrasound, but to actually watch a form manipulating my tummy is incredible. I can touch with my hand and know that I'm feeling my baby. More and more, I sense that I am only a vessel for Your work. There is a part of me, and a part of my husband, but the design and creation are Yours. This child already has a mind of its own, separate from me, and fashioned by You.

I praise You for this amazing miracle. Each day testifies that You are continuing to develop and mature our precious one. I find myself growing anxious now, trying to imagine a face to match the curves and feet strong enough to kick. I know that these next weeks will be a time of rapid growth. The baby will gain weight. The lungs will fully develop. I ask for Your continued protection. Let my baby grow stronger each day. Keep her safely inside until the time is perfect. I eagerly await the unveiling of Your wonder. Thank You for working in me.

AMEN

The LORD made you . . . And formed you from the womb.

— Isaiah 44:2 NAS

GRANDMA HELENE

DEAR GOD,

As this pregnancy progresses, my sentimental feelings increase. I want to look at my own baby book, read the cards sent to my parents, feel the lock of my baby hair, and read about my first words. Thirty-five years ago, I was carried out to meet the world in a little pink dress with white lace and embroidery. Mama framed that dress and it hangs in my bedroom.

I still have my mama to tell me stories and to make sweet gowns for my babies, but Paul's mother is already gone. I have the blankets that carried Paul and little shoes that warmed his feet, but there's so much I'd like to ask her. How did she feel during pregnancy? What was her labor like? How did she prepare for Paul's arrival? I'm sad that my children won't know her in person and that I didn't get to know her better.

Help us to teach our children that the strength of their father came from the strength of his mother. They won't meet her until heaven, but the value of her life will impact many generations in our family. Thank You for the legacy of faith she left us. Thank You for the great memories we have and the lessons she taught. Thank You that she taught Paul about You and modeled the love and perseverance of Christ. May our new family bring honor to her work and commitment.

Thank You for the godly heritage of grand-parents, both here and in heaven, who began the traditions we'll build on. Thank You for loving us through them. In Jesus name,

AMEN

I have been reminded of your sincere faith, which first lived in your grandmother Lois and in your mother Eunice and, I am persuaded, now lives in you also.

— 2 Timothy 1:5

Precious in the sight of the LORD is the death of his saints.

— Psalm 116:15

153

ENCOURAGE ONE ANOTHER

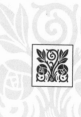

LORD JESUS,

A friend's wife joked it was easy to spot me because, "You look like you're going to pop." She was trying to be funny. I laughingly agreed. But I thought about her words for days. I know she intended no harm, but her words left me feeling discouraged. Then, a lady from Ireland told me, "You must be having a girl. Your tummy looks trim and you're carrying so tidy." The soothing words of encouragement—even from the lips of a stranger, they are sweet. I didn't know I was needy until she walked away and her words remained to nourish me. How can two women look at the same huge belly and respond with such contrasting pronouncements?

And yet, from these two, I have learned a lesson—that encouragement begins in the heart of the beholder. I've spoken to many pregnant women, without thinking of their emotional needs. I could have ministered to those needs if I had consciously chosen to encourage. We choose what to do with our thoughts. We decide whether our words will inspire or dishearten.

Lord, please make me an encourager. Give me eyes to see good and lips that speak love. Let me instinctively know how to inspire and build up. Don't let me trample a tender heart. Remind me how weak we all really are. Each one of us needs cheerleaders and fans. I want to choose everyday to support and applaud. The race is a hard go all alone.

Thank You for the lesson about encouragement. Let me grow in this area to Your glory. Everyday, make me more like You. I love You, Jesus.

AMEN

Encourage one another daily, as long as it is called Today.

— Hebrews 3:13

Confident in Christ

My Father,

I want to be a great mom. I'm excited by the challenges ahead and motivated to learn. I want to pour all of me into every day, and at the end of my life, I want to know that I gave everything. I don't want to hold back because of unwarranted fears. And I don't want to miss the reason You put me here. The years speed by and I never want to look back with remorse or regret.

Lord, I want to be a mommy You're proud of—one that loves with great energy. I want my kids to light up when we're together. I want to add to them and never take away from what they could be.

I want to give them grace and the freedom to try. I want to learn how to care for their hearts.

But, You know I am untrained and unskilled. I entered into motherhood with great aspirations and little understanding. I would hesitate, except I know that You can provide everything I need. You will give wisdom, knowledge, and common sense. To be an excellent mom only requires that I walk with You. Father, I commit to depend on You daily. I will talk to You and read from Your Word. I will come to You before I make decisions. I will seek You for strength and endurance.

I'm excited and ready to go. I'm confident because I know You are with me. I joyfully give thanks for the adventure that lies ahead. May all my efforts bear fruit and bring You glory. In the name of Jesus,

AMEN

We have not stopped praying for you and asking God to fill you with the knowledge of his will through all spiritual wisdom and understanding. And we pray this in order that you may live a life worthy of the Lord and may please him in every way: bearing fruit in every good work, growing in the knowledge of God, being strengthened with all power according to his glorious might so that you may have great endurance and patience, and joyfully giving thanks to the Father.

— Colossians 1:9–12

THE GIFT OF A CHILD

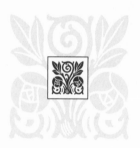

DEAR LORD OF OUR FUTURE,

Already people have begun to ask, "Is this it? Are you ready to do it again? How many children do you want?" I find myself unprepared to respond. I have been so focused on just getting through this pregnancy, that I haven't even tried to process the future. My sights are totally set on one path— staying healthy, getting up everyday, pressing on, and getting this baby here. After that, the Lord will have to direct.

I would imagine almost any woman, in the middle of a miserable day, might yell out loud, "I never, ever want to do this again." I've had several of those days, and they aren't great advertisements for pregnancy. Then, out of nowhere, a day will pop up that's calm and sentimental. My heart is peaceful, and I'm proud to be pregnant. On one of those days, I'd do it again in a minute.

Father, I already treasure the gift growing within me. I know that to hold my child will truly be a reward. In time we will have a full quiver to share our lives with. But for now, I'm sure that this one, this special chosen one, will fill our hours and our hearts with joy beyond measure. We'll trust You for the future and for the dimensions of our quiver. Give us the wisdom to know when it's full.

And so, when those uncomfortable questions come, let me respond with grace, "We'll treasure one gift at a time." I look forward to beholding the fruit You have begun in my womb. Thank You, kind Lord.

AMEN

Behold, children are a gift of the LORD; The fruit of the womb is a reward. Like arrows in the hand of a warrior, So are the children of one's youth. How blessed is the man whose quiver is full of them.

— Psalm 127:3–5 NAS

JOY IN THE TRIALS

DEAR LORD JESUS,

Each month brings more trials than I had anticipated. At first it was the nausea—trying to work, and smile when you feel sick as a dog. Then came the fatigue. I felt like I could barely drag through the day before heading back into bed. There was a lull for awhile when my energy returned and I had to remind myself I was pregnant. But these last three months, no one has had to remind me. My body has fallen apart. My spirit is anxious and fragile. My emotions are a mess.

Besides all the big stuff, even little things feel like trials when you're pregnant. I've stopped wearing shoes I'll have to bend over and tie. Forget socks, they're too tight on my ankles. Hauling groceries into the house does me in. I've decided all those trips to the potty should qualify as calisthenics. Thinking about preparing a meal requires an extra dispensation of grace. And the laundry, well, reaching into the dryer for that last lonely sock, whacks out my back every time. Each endeavor requires so much effort.

Lord, I ask for renewed perseverance—the ability to go on when I'd rather fall down. Thank You for the people who are walking beside me—my husband, my mother, my friends. Their love and support fuel my strength. Thank You for each trial and each lesson. Lord, I pray for the blessings that come from maturity. And in this time, this incredibly trying time, it is a privilege to consider it joy. Because of You, I press on and choose to be glad.

AMEN

Consider it pure joy, my brothers, whenever you face trials of many kinds, because you know that the testing of your faith develops perseverance. Perseverance must finish its work so that you may be mature and complete, not lacking anything.
— James 1:2–4

Blessed is the man who perseveres under trial, because when he has stood the test, he will receive the crown of life that God has promised to those who love him.
— James 1:12

SIMPLIFY

OH MERCIFUL GOD,

I fall before You this afternoon, tired of all the clutter in my life. Too many good things have stolen the quality of my days. My education, my ministry, my writing, my family, my pregnancy, my husband . . . each one a treasure, but all together, overwhelming. I have become a great big cyclone of unfocused energy blown to and fro by the tyranny of the urgent.

I know that all the mayhem in my life keeps me from walking according to Your will. I lay my treasures before You and beg You to begin ordering my steps. What is most important? Where can I simplify? Some wear exhaustion like a badge of godliness, but I don't believe there is anything noble about a life that is spinning. As much as I bristle at the overly busy, I confess that I have unwittingly joined their ranks. I find no pleasure in boasting about how much I have to do. I yearn for a life that bears Your imprint—days of simple enjoyment and relationships grounded in love.

More than anything else, I do want to act justly, love mercy, and walk humbly with my God. Teach me how to let these principles supersede any other aspirations. Show me what "simplify" will look like for me. To wait any longer is to waste more days apart from You, immersed in the clutter.

Thank You for the truth of Your Word, that shouts to me and pulls me back. What You require is what I want. Bless You, God. I love You.

AMEN

He has showed you, O man, what is good.
And what does the LORD require of you? To act
justly and to love mercy and to walk humbly
with your God.

— Micah 6:8

BABY SHOWER

DEAR GOD,

This day has been such a blessing. Thank You, Lord, for Your goodness. So many came to rejoice with me about our baby, and their outpourings of love still cover me. Sitting with my circle of friends chased all my fears away and filled my heart with gladness.

Today I'm not lonely, or afraid, or anxious because I've been strengthened by the people who love me, inspired by their stories to press on, and edified by their prayers. Why have I tried to plod through so many days alone when all the time I've been surrounded by such wonderful friends?

Lord, pour out your blessings on my sisters. Return to them many-fold the kindness they have shown to me. Thank You for the home where we gathered and all the laughter we shared. Thank You for the hands that cleaned and prepared each thoughtful detail—balloons, flowers, petite fours and munchies, a corsage and favors. Thank You for the gifts for our baby—clothes, keepsakes, handmade quilts—things we'll cherish for a lifetime. And thank You especially for the tender time of prayer. What a comfort to listen as each woman prayed for me and for our child. I am humbled and very grateful.

Today You have truly showered me with Your love. I have been hugged by You through my friends, and I rejoice in Your goodness. My heart overflows with gratitude for all You have done on our behalf. Bless my dear friends with the same lavish love that they have given. I give You praise and thank You.

AMEN

Rejoice with those who rejoice.
— Romans 12:15

RESTLESS SLEEP

LORD,

Pregnancy is beginning to take its toll. The day drains my resources, and night fails to replenish. Sleep has become miserable. My exhausted body is screaming for rest, but the person inside won't cooperate.

The ritual of bedtime has quickly grown old. A mountain of pillows stuffed at every angle for maximum support and comfort. A blanket thrown on and off—off and on, depending on the temperature of my toes. A baby that already wants to play at night, kicking and probably laughing out loud, knowing that mama is tired of this game. A heavy body that is relieved for a moment, then groans under the weight of my cargo. Aching everything. My hair even hurts. Bones that fall out of joint in a turn. A bladder that wails at the slightest jolt and must be quickly attended. Up and down. Side to side. This ship isn't easy to steer.

Morning finds me frazzled; still longing for rest that never came. I want to cry. Nobody can help me but You. I know that in time I won't even remember how it felt to be so out of whack. But for tonight, dear Jesus, I need peace. Settle my body, calm all my fears, and when I lie down, bring sleep—blessed sleep.

When I wake in the night, remind me to set my thoughts on You—the God of all power and wisdom, Who never slumbers. Your care for us is constant and never ending. Because You are the God of Comfort and because You are always with me, I can pray in Your powerful name.

AMEN

When you lie down, you will not be afraid;
when you lie down, your sleep will be sweet.
— Proverbs 3:24

BE STILL

LORD ALMIGHTY,

Everything's ready. The nursery is done. Little clothes fill the chest of drawers and hang in the closet. The car seat waits patiently. I have completed my "to-do" lists, but all the while I've had this nagging feeling that I'm forgetting something. I've finally realized that in the blur of activity, I've neglected to spend time with You—worshipping with a still mind and a reverent heart.

This child I am carrying deserves a mommy who is spiritually strong—a woman who walks with God and listens to His leading. This baby needs a mommy who remembers the importance of being still in Your presence.

Come, meet with me in the midst of my need, and fill me up, I pray. I'm not very good at being still, but I yearn for the growth that comes from that time with You. When I'm walking with You, I'm not flighty or jittery—the world doesn't get on my nerves and my cynical heart becomes a heart of compassion. My patience is multiplied. And the reward is a more godly woman. I think I act more like You after I've spent time with You. That's what I want, yet I've let busyness rule my days.

Thank You for letting me start over time and time again. Thank You for forgiving my forgetfulness and for leading me back into Your presence. Please keep me from wandering away. I want many days to be still and truly know You as my God. I want the power of Your presence to transform me from within and make my life a blessing to those around me. Because You alone are worthy of my praise,

AMEN

Be still and know that I am God.
— Psalm 46:10

Preview Contractions

Oh Lord,

Whew—what was that? The pain nearly doubled me over. It rose up from deep in my tummy and hung around for a while. I think I even stopped breathing. Was that Braxton Hicks? The preview contractions? Well, I had certainly been wondering what they felt like. It's a little exciting to experience a real pain, but, at the same time, it reminds me that serious business is on the way.

Just sampling this tiny bit of labor, reminds me how afraid I really am. I don't know if I'm scared of the pain, or terrified about how I'll react. I want to be strong and courageous, but fear that I'll fall down and cry. I know me, and when hormones take over, any emotion is conceivable. I could be tough as nails and endure with grace, or I could melt into a puddle and wail. I know that millions have gone before me, but I'm afraid of my unavoidable turn.

Lord, I already need courage, and pretty soon I'll need more. I don't have any badges for bravery; I'm truly scared half to death. My spirit missed the call to adventure. To think of giving birth frightens me right to my core. The only comfort I possess is the assurance that You will be with me as You always have been.

I will trust in Your promise to sustain me and my little one. When fear overtakes me, I will put my hand in Yours. I will go bravely because You go with me. If perfect love casts out all fear, please love all my fears away. In the strong name of Jesus, I pray.

AMEN

My body is racked with pain, pangs seize me, like those of a woman in labor.

— Isaiah 21:3

Have I not commanded you? Be strong and courageous. Do not be terrified; do not be discouraged, for the LORD your God will be with you wherever you go.

— Joshua 1:9

TREASURE TO PONDER

I've been praying for your baby.

This child will be blessed to have you both as parents.

Are you ready for more joy than you can imagine?

It'll all be worth it, I promise.

Where God gives, God provides.

*The sweetest days I ever knew,
were the tender first days with my baby.*

*The hardest thing you've ever done will bring
you the greatest joy you'll ever know.*

Pray for your baby.

You will blink and these days will be gone. Drink deeply.

You will be a wonderful mommy.

Keep having children, I wish I'd had more.

Write down what you're thinking and praying.

Take one more trip. Go on one more date.
Your life will never be the same again.

Pregnant women are incredibly beautiful.

A baby was the best thing that ever happened to me.

We can't wait to meet who's inside there.

Thank You, God, for friends and family and strangers, who's expressions of joy and words of advice, give us so many treasures to ponder. May we take them to heart and reflect on their truth. Thank You for sending all of their blessings. In the name of Your Son, Who filled His mother's heart with treasure,

AMEN

Mary treasured up all these things and
pondered them in her heart.

— Luke 2:19

Due Date Anxiety

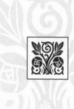

Awesome God,

People ask me again and again, "When are you due?" I give some vague answer and finally declare, "Only God really knows for sure." I count forward and backward, and give it my best guess. Am I in my ninth month or my fortieth week, or is that more like ten months? Everyone else is a great guesser too. *Looks like you've dropped . . . Got your bags packed, it could be any day now?*

And then there's this baby, with a mind of her own. *That baby will come when she's ready.* None of my babies ever come when they're ready. We always have to go in and get them. They get ready, then hang out to dawdle and primp. They get bigger and bigger—so big they barely fit through the door. We drag them into the world kicking and screaming, telling them our patience has worn thin—enough already.

The only thing I know for sure about due dates and babies is that my thoughts are not Your thoughts, and my ways are not Your ways. I'd choose convenience over late-night every time. Sometime after lunch, about mid-afternoon. A few pains and then a delivery. Everyone forewarned and in their place. Dad home from his trip. My mom right beside me. A month of dinners in the freezer. Laundry done for the week. Bags packed and gas in the car.

But where's my sense of adventure? I can't wait to see how Your plan unfolds. Until then, I am resting in the wisdom of Your thoughts, and trusting in the certainty of Your ways. By Your mercy, I will be ready when You are. I love You.

AMEN

"For my thoughts are not your thoughts, neither are your ways my ways," declares the LORD.
— Isaiah 55:8

175

BUILDING A NEST

LORD,

Something incredible is going on with me. There is a sense of urgency about preparations. Things must be done—*everything* must be done, and now. I have a list for me, a list for my husband, and extras for anyone who wants to pitch in. I have energy that has never existed and a burning desire to accomplish minuscule tasks. This must be nesting. If this is common with most pregnant women, then I guess it's a designed response— something You deemed necessary and important to include in the pregnancy package.

I'm wide awake by early in the morning and stay up well past my usual collapse time. I'm a whirlwind of accomplishment. Every sock drawer has been rearranged. The closets have been sorted. The baseboards are scrubbed. The cupboards have been stocked. Baby clothes are washed. Newborn diapers have been purchased. The diaper bag is packed. I am actually finding pleasure in thinking of new chores to do. I might even start working on our tax returns. The longer I act like this, the more I believe this is the real me—superwoman about to become supermom.

But something tells me this season is fleeting. I have been with too many new moms. They don't even brush their teeth anymore. They wear the same old sweatpants for weeks. Nesting is long past and survival is in. They could kick themselves for ever working into the night without reason.

Lord, thank You for this time of achievement. It has felt good to get so many things done. I look forward to the child who has caused all this commotion. I am ready and waiting.

AMEN

A wife of noble character who can find? She is worth far more than rubies. She selects wool and flax and works with eager hands. She is like the merchant ships, bringing her food from afar. She gets up while it is still dark. She sets about her work vigorously; her arms are strong for her tasks . . . her lamp does not go out at night.

— Proverbs 31:10, 13–15, 17–18

FEAR IN THE LAST DAYS

MY FATHER,

Only a few weeks to go. My doctor and I have talked through scenarios. When to call her. What to do. Should we induce? Should we wait a little longer? Maybe another ultrasound just to check. Then there are the technical things. The baby hasn't turned yet. Am I measuring too big? Low iron. High blood pressure. Dilating. Effacing.

All these months of normal pregnancy and now everything's crazy at the end. A routine delivery seemed scary enough. And with just minor complications, I've become anxious. My mind writes emergency dramas. *Baby born in blizzard. Baby born at the grocery store. Baby delivered by four year-old.*

What is going on with me? I trust in You. How does this garbage get into my head?

I know that You will uphold me, yet I'm dwelling on *ifs*. *If* this or *if* that? *Ifs* make you loony and I know better. Please take all these bizarre *ifs* away. Let me process only valid concerns. Give me calm thoughts and a confident heart. I need courage to face whatever comes. Revoke the temptation to let my mind wander. Keep me focused on Your strong right hand that upholds.

No one can relieve my fears like You. My comfort is that You are with me. You go to the hospital before me. You prepare each instrument used. You intervene to protect. You give wisdom where there is lack. And above all this, You do miracles. What more could I need than the Almighty God who has promised to always be with me?

I will take a deep breath and rest in Your strength. Your promises restore my sanity. Prayer brings great peace. Thank You, dear Father.

AMEN

So do not fear, for I am with you; do not be dismayed, for I am your God. I will strengthen you and help you; I will uphold you with my righteous right hand.

— Isaiah 41:10

MY ACHING BODY

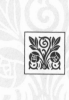

LORD,

How is it that so many women work right up until the day they deliver? I have three weeks to go and I'm about to come to a complete stand-still. My body aches almost all day long, and the night brings little relief. Heartburn and indigestion. Nasal congestion and a stuffy head. Headaches and dizzy spells. Persistent fatigue and sleeplessness. Leg cramps and a tender back. It just keeps coming.

I couldn't possibly get any bigger. My tummy feels as tight as a drum. My clothes feel awful. Every chore requires a mental pep rally just to motivate this body to move. I can only sit for a little while and then I need to stand up. I huff across the room to shake out my bones, and in just a few minutes, I need to lie down. Lying down is fine for awhile, and then one whole side starts to ache.

Lord, I feel like a mess. My emotions have worn thin. I'm tired of feeling lousy. Tears spring up easily. I know that only You can sustain me. I don't want to be a total grouch these last few weeks. Please lift me above the discomfort, and let me find joy in these days. I am counting on You to provide stamina where I have none. I am trusting You to carry me to delivery. Help me to hear Your voice above the aches and pains—Your whispers of comfort and hope.

Thank You for Your love and faithfulness to this mommy-to-be. With my heart focused on Your infinite goodness, I pray in Your strong name.

AMEN

I am poured out like water, and all my bones are out of joint.

— Psalm 22:14

181

HELP FROM HEAVEN

LORD,

I have prayed many prayers about my weakness. I have come to You full of anxiety and fear. This journey has made me weary. My strength is depleted. Just last night I asked You for help . . . something or someone to shore me up until I can get to the end. Thank You for sending the entire cavalry.

Thank You for the first wave of troops. The folks who've offered to sit with our children. The families on standby to come in the night. The friends who've called to ask what they can do. Lucille and her great apple pies. Please bless each one of these givers.

But this afternoon, You sent the best of the battalion. The surprise knock at our door belonged to my parents. From twelve hours away, they drove in to help us get ready for the baby. It felt like a dream to fall into their arms and hug them tight. I am so thankful they're here. Please honor their willingness to serve You and love me.

I realize that each one represents the help I had prayed for. You heard my cries and You answered. I am very humbled. I know that You love me and I think I pray believing, until You answer so loudly. I realize that I barely understand what it means to believe. I trust, but only with human trust. I love, but with the flawed love of a sinner. Thank You for hearing and answering my prayers.

Your daughter hears tonight. I hear You shouting Your love for me. I love You too. In the great name of Your Son,

AMEN

God is not unjust; he will not forget your work
and the love you have shown him as you have
helped his people and continue to help them.
— Hebrews 6:10

183

THE END TIMES

LORD,

This should be my last week of waiting, and I'm not sure I can hold it together. I have stepped beyond *out of whack* into *totally wigged out.* My emotions are so frayed I can hardly make polite conversation in the check-out line. Someone asked me today, "When are you due?" It was all I could do to keep from bursting into tears before squeaking out a feeble, "Anytime now."

My husband looks at me and says, "What can I do?" hoping for something to fix. There is nothing to report except that I am miserable inside and out, from head to toe, and all around the middle. Every little pregnancy annoyance has meshed together and exploded, making me a walking, talking, crying version of the tribulation. Doom and gloom. Pain and suffering. Lots of weeping, wailing, and gnashing of teeth.

I washed my contact lens down the drain this morning, thinking it was in my eye the whole time. No wonder everything was blurry. Later, I found the cereal in the refrigerator and the peanut butter in the freezer. I drove by my exit twice, both ways, on the way home from the doctor. What's happening to me? I'm a mental mess. I'm almost afraid of myself. I'm sure if tested, I'd be certifiably crazy today.

These are the last days, and I am incredibly ready for You to deliver me from myself. Oh Lord, please interrupt my frustration and hold me tightly. Hear my cries and rescue my weary body. Fear has given way completely to desperation. I collapse into Your arms. I love You.

AMEN

May my cry come before you, O LORD; give me understanding according to your word. May my supplication come before you; deliver me according to your promise.

— Psalm 119:169–170

A Baby Dedication

Dear Lord of Life,

Even before birth, and the first breaths of life, I dedicate our baby to You. I want her to be wholly consecrated and set aside for You.

As parents, we commit to raise this new one in righteousness and grace. We will love each other deeply. We will speak of You, and pray to You, and look to You in our home. We will fellowship with other believers and introduce this baby to Your disciples. We will treasure Your Word and give it honor. We will seek out and welcome the lost. We will forgive and ask for forgiveness. We will practice kindness. We will love the poor and abandoned. We will live under the covering of grace. We will give away the grace we've received. We will fear You as Almighty and trust You as Savior.

We come with uncertainties, sin, and shortcomings—all the things that could keep us from trying. When we lose our way or fail in our efforts, remind us to run toward the cross. Not on our own, but by Your strength, we commit to be godly parents.

We intentionally lay out treasure before You; returning the gift You have given. We know that Your goodness is greater than ours. We trust in Your wisdom more than our own. We have faith in You, not ourselves.

With reverence and devotion, we dedicate our child-yet-unseen to You; the Lord God Almighty; Wondrous and Awesome; Esteemed and Adored. May this sweet one honor You all the days of her life. By grace, You will make us parents, and from grace, we pray in Your name.

AMEN

From birth I was cast upon you; from my mother's womb you have been my God.
— Psalm 22:10

I prayed for this child, and the LORD has granted me what I asked of him. So now I give him to the LORD. For his whole life he will be given over to the Lord.
— 1 Samuel 1:27–28

187

Fear of Cesarean

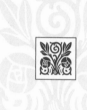

Lord,

The possibility of a cesarean birth seems to be increasing. I am completely caught off guard. I know that anything can happen, but I didn't expect a baby who can't find her way out. The doctor says wait another week or so, maybe everything will change. Meanwhile, I have been reading about C-sections. I think I have more information than I wanted.

Only You know what the future holds. And You also know what a big chicken I am. Surgery. Yuck. I don't want to think about incisions, anesthesia, stitches, abdominal pain, and long days of recuperating. I had made other plans. I was going to be in and out in a day or so, back in the loop in two weeks. And we both know I don't have a very high tolerance for pain.

Only You could listen with such patience and quietly reassure me that the future is Yours. No surprises. Nothing You can't handle. An easy task for an Almighty God. You are the master of this miracle. The Creator who knows better than best. Please forgive my impulse to panic.

While I may feel unprepared and doubt my resilience, I will not doubt Your judgment. However You choose to deliver this child, I will trust in Your wisdom. I will also trust You for the courage I lack. Keep me focused on the precious reward that awaits the end of this work. Because You are abundant where I am inadequate . . . because You are omnipotent where I am feeble . . . because You are Creator and I am created . . . I worship and exalt You.

AMEN

But you, be strong and do not lose courage, for there is reward for your work.
— 2 Chronicles 15:7 NAS

189

ARE YOU STILL HERE?

DEAR GOD,

Everyone is full of suggestions. Spend the afternoon riding over speed bumps. Go to the mall and walk this baby out. Eat lots of spicy food for lunch. One teaspoon of castor oil would get us a baby by tonight. A little dancing or jumping might do the trick. The recommendations are endless, and I'm about ready to start trying a few.

Life is all about waiting, but these last days have been one huge concentrated lesson. I do want to wait on You. I want this baby in Your time. But my heart grows faint, my patience runs thin, and I want to shout, "Could You hurry this up?" I need the strength to wait with renewed endurance and peace. I know this baby is coming out one way or the other, and I trust that You have appointed the very hour and minute. In just a few days, my thirst will be quenched and my hunger will be fed. I will be holding the good thing that has come to those who wait.

Until then, Lord, I will turn to You daily for fresh patience. I will fix my eyes on the treasure ahead. I will sing to this child. I will pray for my baby. Anticipation makes the gift all the better. I am bursting with anticipation. I look forward to the day I'll always remember . . . a day I'll recount until death . . . a day that will be packed with vivid memories . . . I look forward to the birthday of my child. I take heart because You are my Lord.

AMEN

Wait for the LORD; be strong and take heart and wait for the LORD.

— Psalm 27:14

THE PLAN TO INDUCE

LORD,

My doctor thinks we'll have to induce to get
this baby here safely. My tummy is measuring two
weeks too big and the last ultrasound estimates that
the baby already weighs about nine pounds . . .
Nine Pounds!

I don't know why I feel hesitant about
induction. Maybe it's the idea of IV's and drugs that
bothers me. Maybe it's all those conversations ringing
in my ears, "That baby'll come when it gets good and
ready." Maybe it's my fear of the unknown.

We have an appointment for next Tuesday at
dawn. I keep hoping something will happen before

then. Feel free to interrupt our plans and bring this baby sooner! I could have never imagined hoping for pain. But that's how I feel. I'm ready to feel pain . . . good hard pain about five minutes apart. Only You could prepare a woman to want to hurt.

Despite my fears, and my reluctance, I place my trust completely in You—once again! You, in Your sovereignty and wisdom . . . You, Who oversees all things . . . You will work through the doctors and my body to bring about good. The good is that, one way or another, I will be holding my baby by next Tuesday. That promise is more than good; it's awesome.

I have seen the way You have worked things for good in my past. I believe that no matter how my labor begins, You will continue to work all things for good. All of my hope is in You. I do love You so.

AMEN

And we know that in all things God works for the good of those who love him, who have been called according to his purpose.

— Romans 8:28

HERE WE GO!

PRECIOUS LORD WHO WATCHES OVER ME,

The doctor says the day is approaching. Today or tomorrow we should have a baby. Wow. After all this time, it's finally here. I feel like a kid standing in line to ride a roller coaster. I'm eager with anticipation and scared to death at the same time. I look at what's before me in awe—excited to know that it will soon be my turn . . . anxious to experience the thrill once again.

I'm giddy, chatting, and puttering around, trying not to think about it. It's like that same wait for the roller coaster . . . you want the line to move fast, but then you feel sick when it's time to strap in. You want to go, but you don't want to go. I definitely want to go. Actually, I couldn't be more ready. Nine months have prepared me well . . . let's do it! I only get to do this a few times in my lifetime.

Lord, I lift up my eyes to You. I know that my help will come from You. You will watch over me and protect me. You will not slumber or sleep. You will keep me from harm. You will safeguard my baby. Your mercies will be tender and compassionate. I bless You, Lord. You have not looked away. You attend me with great care and compassion.

I will be brave and peaceful, because I depend on You. Keep me close and never let me go. I do not walk alone because of You. Both now and forever-more, I love You.

AMEN

I lift up my eyes to the hills—where does my help come from? My help comes from the LORD, the Maker of heaven and earth. He will not let your foot slip—he who watches over you will not slumber; indeed he who watches over Israel will neither slumber nor sleep. The LORD watches over you—the LORD is your shade at your right hand; the sun will not harm you by day, nor the moon by night. The LORD will keep you from all harm—he will watch over your life; the LORD will watch over your coming and going both now and forevermore.

— Psalm 121

THE TIME HAS COME

Paperwork.
ID bracelets. An IV drip. Ouch. Tummy belts.
The soft lull of a heartbeat.
Nurse Susan. Dr. Jones is on call.
One nervous husband. Goofy jokes.
Nurses chatter outside. Ice chips. Cold feet.
Mama's here.
Tightness in my tummy.
Hours. Real pain.
Dr. Carducci. Tears. An epidural, please.
Progress and predictions.
Visitors. Prayers.
Many hours. Lots of pain.
It's time. A flurry of activity.
Method breathing. Cheers.
She's here . . . praise God, she's here.

FATHER,

Birth is the most amazing thing I have ever experienced in my whole life. You are amazing. I will never do anything more worthy. Thank You.

AMEN

There is a time for everything, and a season for every activity under heaven: a time to be born.
— Ecclesiastes 3:1–2

While they were there, the time came for the baby to be born, and she gave birth to her firstborn, a son.
— Luke 2:6–7

WE DID IT!

LORD,

I did it! I mean—we did it! I gave birth to a child, our child, our daughter! The whole day was exhilarating, even through the hardest pain and rivers of tears, I look back at the adventure as the greatest joy I've ever known. I could have never imagined that one incredibly hard day would be so worth it. I'd march right back in there today and say, "Give it to me double," for the reward of this precious newborn child.

Childbirth has to be one of Your best miracles. What has been hidden is revealed and in a blink, a perfect person is here, crying, breathing, and sucking her thumb. I am so honored to have been the vessel for Your work. I am humbled to think that we worked together to bring this child into the world. I'd like to take credit for this angel, but when I look at her, I know that I had nothing to do with it. Her creator is Almighty God.

I have waited all my life to know this experience, and I feel so proud. I still can't believe I gave birth and lived to tell about it. The biggest chicken this side of heaven did something really brave, and it was awesome! I have never known more joy than I do this very moment.

You are worthy of all glory and honor and praise. You are more than amazing. You are magnificent, and I honor You with my joy. My heart runs over with praise for Your greatness. From my full and overflowing heart I extol You. I love You.

AMEN

A woman giving birth to a child has pain because her time has come; but when her baby is born she forgets the anguish because of her joy that a child is born into the world.

— John 16:21

A Grateful Heart

Glorious God,

Anna Grace Nicole. She is exceeding abundantly beyond all that we could have ever asked or hoped for. My heart surely stopped the first time I saw her—she takes my breath away. I have felt her move all these months, imagined how she might look, and dreamed of this day, but holding her in my arms leaves me speechless. I am full of emotion—waves of tears and laughter wash over me.

I have prayed believing and expecting that You would answer my prayers, yet now that You have, I am moved by the depth of Your love for me. I love You with all my feeble human love, but nothing about me is worthy of this wonderful gift. To hold my child, is to hold the very essence of Your grace.

Now, at the end of pregnancy, there is a new beginning. I am the mother of Anna Grace. Please find me faithful to seek Your guidance and wisdom. Teach me how to love my daughter well. Make of me a godly parent. Empower me with the presence of Your Holy Spirit. Hold me close to You. Keep me praying.

Our family celebrates this birth, but even more, we celebrate Your goodness to us. Your mighty love has come down in abundance as we look lovingly into her eyes, caress her tender new skin, and hold her close enough to feel her breath. Her very presence proves that You exist. Who could look into the eyes of such a miracle and doubt the reality of God? I shall never doubt.

I love You and praise You with all my being.

AMEN

Now to Him who is able to do exceeding abundantly beyond all that we ask or think, according to the power that works within us, to Him be the glory in the church and in Christ Jesus to all generations forever and ever. Amen.
— Ephesians 3:20–21 NAS

Scripture Index

Genesis 1:27-28	The Next Generation
Genesis 3:16	Fear of the Pain
Exodus 1:20-21	My Doctor
Numbers 6:24-26	A Peaceful Countenance
Joshua 1:9	Preview Contractions
Joshua 24:14-15	A Household of Faith
1 Samuel 1:10	For Those Who Still Wait
1 Samuel 1:27-28	A Baby Dedication
2 Chronicles 15:7	Fear of Cesarean
Job 10:8-12	The Ultrasound
Psalm 10:14	Baby Jasmine
Psalm 22:10	A Baby Dedication
Psalm 22:14	My Aching Body
Psalm 27:14	Are You Still Here?
Psalm 30:4-5	Many Tears
Psalm 33:18, 20-22	Miscarriage Fears
Psalm 34:7	Guardian Angels
Psalm 40:5	My Blessings
Psalm 46:10	Be Still
Psalm 56:3-4	No Movement
Psalm 61:1-2	A Faint Heart
Psalm 78:5-7	A Journal
Psalm 91:11	Guardian Angels
Psalm 103:1	Thank You
Psalm 113:9	For Those Who Still Wait
Psalm 115:12-15	A Nursery Blessing
Psalm 116:15	Grandma Helene
Psalm 119:169-170	The End Times
Psalm 121	Here We Go!
Psalm 127:3-5	The Gift of a Child
Psalm 139:13-16	Waiting to Know
Psalm 141:3	Guard My Mouth
Proverbs 3:5	A Disabled Child
Proverbs 3:24	Restless Sleep
Proverbs 4:1-4	My Husband, a Father
Proverbs 4:5	Forgetful
Proverbs 6:20-23	A Godly Heritage
Proverbs 15:22	Much Advice about Everything
Proverbs 17:17	A Pregnant Friend

Proverbs 17:22	The Heartbeat
Proverbs 20:18	Much Advice about Everything
Proverbs 21:23	Guard My Mouth
Proverbs 22:1	Our Baby's Name
Proverbs 24:3-4	A House Blessing
Proverbs 27:7	Cravings
Proverbs 31:10-18	Building a Nest
Ecclesiastes 3:1-2	The Time Has Come
Ecclesiastes 4:9-10	A Pregnant Friend
Ecclesiastes 5:12	Blessed Sleep
Song of Songs 5:16	My Husband, My Friend
Isaiah 21:3	Preview Contractions
Isaiah 40:28-31	Renewed Strength
Isaiah 41:10	Fear in the Last Days
Isaiah 43:18-19	Ready to Mommy
Isaiah 44:2	The Commotion Inside
Isaiah 44.24	In the Womb
Isaiah 49:1	Our Baby's Name
Isaiah 55:8	Due Date Anxiety
Isaiah 66:11	Nursing
Jeremiah 1:5	Baby's Purpose
Jeremiah 29:11	God Shouts
Jeremiah 31:34	My Sin
Lamentations 3:22-23	The Fruit of My Spirit
Micah 6:8	Simplify
Micah 7:19	My Sin
Matthew 5:14-15	The Glow
Matthew 6:9-10	Thy Will Be Done
Matthew 6:22	The Glow
Matthew 6:34	How Many Children?
Matthew 11:28-30	Rest for the Weary
Luke 1:44	The Leap Within
Luke 2:4,5	Great with Child
Luke 2:6-7	The Time Has Come
Luke 2:7	Baby Stuff
Luke 2:19	Treasure to Ponder
Luke 5:16	A Retreat
Luke 12:22-26	Do Not Worry
John 3:16-17	That She Would Believe

John 8:31,32	Strange Teaching
John 16:21	We Did It!
John 17:14-15	A Crooked Generation
Romans 8:28	The Plan to Induce
Romans 12:10	Friends Forever
Romans 12:15	Baby Shower
1 Corinthians 13:7-8	My Child's Will
1 Corinthians 14:33	Confused By Pregnancy
2 Corinthians 1:3-5	God of All Comfort
2 Corinthians 3:5	Feelings of Inadequacy
2 Corinthians 6:14	Baby-In-Law
2 Corinthians 12:9	Weak Days
Galatians 5:22-23	The Fruit of my Spirit
Ephesians 3:20-21	A Grateful Heart
Ephesians 4:29	My Grumpy Self
Ephesians 5:25-26, 28-29	My Husband, My Love
Philippians 2:15	A Crooked Generation
Philippians 2:14-15	Complaining
Philippians 4:6-7	Everyone Else's Story
Philippians 4:19	Baby Stuff
Colossians 1:9-12	Confident in Christ
Colossians 3:13	A Time to Forgive
1 Thessalonians 5:11	The Encourager
2 Timothy 1:5	Grandma Helene
Titus 2:3-4	A Mommy Mentor
Hebrews 3:13	Encourage One Another
Hebrews 6:10	Help from Heaven
Hebrews 10:25	My Church
Hebrews 11:1	Faith Journey
Hebrews 12:1-2	My Sin
Hebrews 13:9	Strange Teaching
James 1:2-4	Joy in the Trials
James 1:12	Joy in the Trials
James 1:16-17	Good and Perfect Gifts
James 1:27	Baby Jasmine
James 5:16	Prayers of the Faithful
1 Peter 5:7	Many Tears
1 John 4:7	A Kindred Spirit

About the Author

Angela Thomas Guffey is a graduate of The University of North Carolina at Chapel Hill and Dallas Theological Seminary. She and her husband Paul live outside Orlando where she is a stay-at-home mom to their four 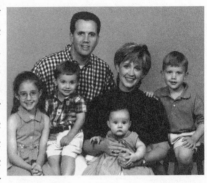 children. She teaches a women's Bible study and is a frequent speaker at women's retreats, conferences, and seminars. *Prayers for Expectant Mothers* was written during her fourth pregnancy.

You can write to Angela via the internet at:
Angela@Worshiphim.com.

Additional copies of this book
are available from
your local bookstore.

Coming Soon
Prayers for New Mothers

Honor Books
Tulsa, Oklahoma